Rehabilitation Nursing
for the Neurological Patient

Marcia Hanak, BSN, MA, CRRN, received her BSN at the University of Arizona and her MA at New York University. During her nursing career she has held a variety of positions in acute care, rehabilitation, and in community health agencies. She is the author of *Patient and Family Education: Teaching Programs for Managing Chronic Disease and Disability* (1986), and the coauthor of *Spinal Cord Injury: An Illustrated Guide for Health Care Professionals* (1983). In addition, she has lectured extensively, edited a nursing manual, written two patient handbooks, a video program, a rehabilitation teaching manual and numerous articles. Prior to assuming her present position as a rehabilitation consultant she served as the clinical coordinator for rehabilitation at Mount Sinai Medical Center in New York City, the Patient Education Coordinator at the Rusk Institute of Rehabilitation Medicine, New York University Medical Center (New York City), and the Spinal Cord Injury Nursing Coordinator, New York University Medical Center.

REHABILITATION NURSING FOR THE NEUROLOGICAL PATIENT

Marcia Hanak, BSN, MA, CRRN

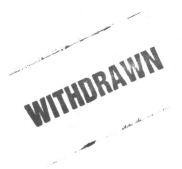

SPRINGER PUBLISHING COMPANY
New York

Springer Publishing Company, Inc.
536 Broadway
New York, NY 10012-3955

92 93 94 95 96 / 5 4 3 2 1

Hanak, Marcia.
    Rehabilitation nursing for the neurological patient / Marcia Hanak.
      p.   cm.
    ISBN 0-8261-7660-7
    1. Neurological nursing.   2. Central nervous system—Diseases—
Patients—Rehabilitation.   3. Mentally handicapped—Rehabilitation.
I. Title.
    [DNLM: 1. Nervous System Diseases—nursing.   2. Nervous System
Diseases—rehabilitation—nurses' instruction.
WY 160 H233r]
RC350.5.H36   1992
610.73'68—dc20
DNLM/DLC
for Library of Congress   91-5189
                                                                CIP

Printed in the United States of America

In memory of my father
who taught me the greatest
lessons of rehabilitation
by the way he lived his life.

Contents

Introduction

Rehabilitation can be defined as a dynamic, evolving process that facilitates physical, psychological, and social reintegration in order to help the person with a disability regain the confidence and ability to successfully manage life's experiences. It does this by:

- promoting self-responsibility, awareness, and motivation;
- promoting the development of physical, social, problem-solving, and coping skills; and by
- encouraging the individual to seek growth producing challenges, to relate to others in a positive, flexible manner, and to engage in health enhancing activities.

A similar description has been used by C. Clark (*Wellness Nursing: Concepts, Theory, Research, and Practice.* New York: Springer, 1986) to define wellness. The fact that these definitions of rehabilitation and wellness can be used interchangeably is a reflection of the interrelationship of the two concepts. The learning process is an essential component of this interrelationship.

The rehabilitation nurse has an integral multifaceted role in facilitating each person's progress toward optimum wellness and successful rehabilitation. This role is not confined to nurses working within rehabilitation facilities. It is assumed by any nurse who works with persons who have neurological disabilities.

This book is designed to serve as a resource to maximize each nurse's effectiveness in this multifaceted role of teacher, coordinator, care provider, counselor, and facilitator. Part I focuses on three of the primary areas of responsibility for the rehabilitation nurse: wellness promotion, patient education, and an understanding of neuroanatomy. These areas are also addressed within the context of each subsequent chapter. Part II reviews the physiology, pathophysiology, and nursing management of problems frequently encountered in neurorehabilitation. Part III reviews the pathophysiology of specific disabilities and the related nursing interventions.

The psychology of rehabilitation, the role of the family, and comprehensive discharge planning are primary aspects of any rehabilitation program. Each of these topics merits an entire book of its own: here, they are addressed from the broader perspectives of ongoing wellness promotion and education activities. In addition, related psychosocial considerations are included in the nursing intervention section of each chapter. Psychosocial and discharge planning references are listed in Appendix I. National resource organizations and phone numbers are listed in Appendix II.

In summary, it is hoped that this book will serve as a useful reference for all nurses working with persons with neurological disabilities, stimulate the reader's desire for further research on the topics presented, and facilitate the nurse–patient interactions that maximize the patient's potential for achieving optimum wellness and successful rehabilitation.

Overview

Wellness Promotion

1

OBJECTIVES

After completing this chapter, the reader will be able to:

- Discuss the differences between health and wellness.
- Describe how a disability may affect a person's ability to achieve optimum wellness.
- Relate health and wellness models and theories to the practice of rehabilitation nursing.
- Discuss cultural values and influences and how these may affect wellness activities.
- Discuss the interventions that can assist the person with a disability in achieving optimum wellness.

INTRODUCTION

Major changes are occurring in health care today. Some of the most significant are a gradual shift from an illness focus to a wellness focus, increased consumer awareness with a corresponding increase in consumer health care decision making and responsibility, and increased funding by government and private companies for prevention and health promotion programs. Knowledge of the concepts of wellness is essential for the rehabilitation nurse, as one of the primary goals of rehabilitation nursing is to help the person with a neurological disability achieve and maintain a high level of wellness.

DEFINITIONS OF HEALTH AND WELLNESS

Health and wellness are not synonymous. Health is defined as a static passive condition, such as "free from disease." In 1947 the World Health Organization (WHO) defined health in broader but still static terms as "a state of complete physical, mental, and social well being and not merely the absence of disease or infirmity." Other definitions of health also convey the notion of a static condition of physical, mental, social, and spiritual well-being (Clark, 1986).

Rather than a static condition, wellness is defined as a dynamic, evolving process reflecting physical, psychological, and social integration and growth within an individual, and an enhanced quality of life. The pursuit of wellness involves self responsibility, awareness, and motivation. A person moves toward wellness by seeking growth-producing challenges, relating to others in a positive and flexible manner, engaging in health enhancing activities, and developing and using effective coping strategies. This person develops and uses problem solving skills, displays a willingness to learn and change, demonstrates a commitment to goals, and feels in control of self and confident of managing life's experiences (Clark, 1986). Because the concept of wellness involves an interrelationship between all dimensions of a person's life, wellness promotion requires a holistic approach that addresses these dimensions and their interrelationships.

Achieving optimum wellness can be a major challenge for persons with neurological disabilities. Rather than experiencing integration and growth in the physical, psychological, and social dimensions of their lives, they are likely to experience major disruptions. In addition, their abilities to use previous problem solving, self-care, and coping skills may be severely compromised and their goals and personal relationships abruptly changed. The rehabilitation nurse plays an integral role in assisting these individuals to identify how their disabilities have affected each dimension of their lives and in learning the problem solving, self-care, and psychosocial skills needed to successfully reintegrate these changed dimensions and achieve optimum wellness.

MODELS AND THEORIES

Several health and wellness models and theories have been selected to demonstrate their holistic focus and their applicability to rehabilitation nursing.

The Eberst health cube model (Eberst, 1984) is a multidimensional approach that emphasizes the importance of focusing on the patient as a whole person. Each health dimension occupies a side of the cube and each dimension has sub-elements. The six dimensions and the related sub-elements are: physical (systemic functioning, fitness, risk behavior, and stress exposure); emotional (self-perception, ability to express feelings appropriately, sexuality, and ability to relate personal values and demonstrate empathy); mental (cognition, adaptation, judgment, coping ability); spiritual (trust, integrity, ethics, feelings of selflessness, and an ability to love and be loved); and vocation (having life goals, advancement, and financial success). Changing any of the sub-elements affects the entire cube, as one sub-element in every dimension is affected. They interact synergistically, with the total effect greater than the sum of two parts taken independently. Making health behavior changes involves considering all six dimensions. This consideration is especially important for individuals with neurological disabilities as they have usually experienced dramatic changes in some or all of these dimensions.

The vulnerability/risk/human response/care model (Shaver, 1985) describes the integrated function of a whole individual from a biopsychosocial view and explains the interaction between the environment and the individual in relation to his/her health status. In this model vulnerability factors are those within an individual that are related to health and wellness such as physiological status, self-concept, and genetic predisposition. Risks are those elements outside the individual that can affect health and wellness. Human response refers to a potential or real change in health status such as pain or grief related to loss of function. Care refers to the assessment and planned intervention designed to effect positive changes in the individual's response to health and wellness promotion, for example health and wellness education and symptom management.

In applying this model to health care planning for the person with a disability it is evident that special considerations are required. In relation to vulnerability factors the individual's physiological status and self-concept will have undergone changes. The risks to health are likely to be increased because of the disability-related physiological changes. Grief related to functional and psychosocial losses and pain related to the neurological dysfunction are frequently encountered human responses. By addressing these biopsychosocial changes the nurse can more effectively implement wellness promotion activities.

In Pender's health promotion model (Pender, 1982), factors such as self-esteem, perceived control, and perceived health status interact with modifying factors such as demographic, interpersonal, and situational variables and perceived barriers to influence the likelihood of change within the individual. All these factors may be altered after a person has sustained a disability. Without proper support and guidance in managing each alteration the individual is likely to have greater difficulty in making the self-care and lifestyle changes required for successful adaptation.

Sr. Callista Roy developed an adaptation model that views man as a biopsychosocial being interacting constantly with a changing environment (Roy, 1984). According to Roy, health can be identified along a health illness continuum and is affected by a variety of environmental stimuli. A positive response to these stimuli requires adaptation. A person with a disability experiences major physiological, self-concept, and role changes that can interfere with his/her ability to adapt. The nurse's role is to assist the individual in developing coping abilities that facilitate adaptation and movement toward optimum health and wellness.

Other health promotion models and theories focus on specific characteristics that can affect a person's health and wellness status. Though these models and theories are helpful in health care planning they may have limited applicability for persons with brain damage as they describe traits and activities associated with higher level cognitive abilities.

Kobasa's theory of hardiness (Kobasa, Maddi, & Zola, 1983) describes persons high in hardiness as demonstrating commitment, control, and being stimulated and challenged by change. People with low levels of hardiness are described as alienated, powerless, and threatened by change. While sustaining a disability is an overwhelming experience for everyone, the person with a low level of hardiness can be expected to have greater difficulty in adjusting than one who has a high level of hardiness. This suggests that special interventions may be required to involve the low hardiness individual in peer group activities and in his/her program planning and to keep scheduling and environmental changes to a minimum.

The theory of self-efficacy (Bandura, 1977) describes high self-efficacy as the ability to organize and mobilize social, cognitive, and behavioral skills and to do these in changing circumstances. A patient with this ability to mobilize skills in a highly stressful rehabilitation setting is more likely to achieve maximum potential.

The type A/B personality construct (Siegel, 1984; Dembroski, MacDougall, Williams, Haney, & Blumenthal, 1985) describes the person with a hostile type A personality as having an increased sympathetic response to environmental stress, an inability to relax, an obsessive involvement with work, an exaggerated sense of time urgency and competition, and a tendency to suppress symptoms of fatigue. Without timely intervention this type of behavior can lead to compromised health and exacerbate health problems following a disability. In contrast, the person with a type B personality has characteristics that are more likely to be health enhancing. These characteristics include a relaxed attitude toward task mastery, an expanded sense of time, and an attunement and responsiveness to fatigue symptoms.

This small sample of health and wellness models and theories serves to illustrate the point that wellness promotion activities require a holistic perspective. Also, it is evident that these models and theories can be readily adapted for use in the rehabilitation setting.

CULTURAL VALUES AND INFLUENCES

Values represent a system of attitudes, ideas, and beliefs that bind individuals together in a common culture. They underlie each person's perception of self in relation to others and the world as a whole, and influence his/her response to wellness promotion activities.

McInerney (1984) uses the following categories of values as a general guide to identify cultural variations. Some of the behaviors associated with these values are discussed for purposes of explanation, not to propose that individual responses can be neatly categorized.

Internal versus external control relates to the degree to which individuals feel they can effect change in their lives. Some cultures support the concept of an internal locus of control in which individuals can effect changes and control their own lives. Persons from this cultural orientation tend to respond well to wellness promotion and independent learning activities. They are likely to be successful at mobilizing personal resources to achieve positive health behaviors. Other cultures feel that external factors control a person's destiny (external locus of control). Individuals with this cultural orientation may be less able to mobilize personal resources as they feel relatively helpless to control the course of their own lives. They are more likely to respond to wellness promotion activities that have clearly defined objectives, are subdivided into easily managed tasks, and provide ongoing reinforcement.

Good versus bad relates to how a culture views human nature. Some cultures believe that a person is basically good and requires few outside rules and regulations. There is an emphasis on personal freedom. An individual with this cultural orientation may have little practice with schedules and goal setting but may respond well to a flexible, individualized wellness promotion program. Other cultures believe that individuals need stringent rules and regulations to guide their behavior. A person with this orientation is likely to have difficulty developing personal priorities and may respond best to group-approved wellness programs.

Open versus closed and "tight versus loose" relates to group norms regarding privacy and the family unit. In some cultures the accepted distance between persons in a social situation is approximately 3 feet. Coming closer or touching without permission is considering a violation. An individual's problems and needs are considered confidential and discussed only in the nuclear family unit. For wellness promotion interventions to be accepted they must be presented in a manner that does not violate the individual's personal boundaries and privacy preferences. In other cultures the accepted distance between persons in a social situation may be only inches. Touching is an integral part of communication. The individual's problems and needs tend to be shared with an extended family unit. Wellness promotion interventions are likely to be more accepted when adaptations are made to incorporate the extended family. However, this can make planning more difficult unless rules are established and one family member is designated as the contact person.

Present versus future relates to a culture's orientation to time. Some groups are future oriented and stress the importance of getting ahead. Persons within these groups tend to live with a sense of time urgency. Often crisis events are the only times they are willing to stop and evaluate their lives and health behaviors. Other cultures are present oriented and less accepting of long-range wellness promotion recommendations. In this case daily learning activities, short-term goals, and frequent positive reinforcement may facilitate acceptance and compliance.

Other factors within a culture that can impact an individual's health and wellness behaviors include specific beliefs about health and illness and special traditions, rituals, and taboos.

NURSING INTERVENTIONS

Learner Assessment

Demographic information including age, marital status, occupation, education level, primary language, and financial status.

Cognitive information including brain disease or injury related impairments, perceived health and wellness information needs and learning priorities, current level of knowledge of health and wellness practices.

Physical information including health history and current health status and practices, musculoskeletal limitations, diminished visual and hearing acuity, reduced tolerance secondary to pain, fatigue, and/or deconditioning.

Psychological information including presence of affective disorders related to brain damage, presence of fear, anxiety, and depression; type and effectiveness of coping style; level of maturity; self-image; personal meaning of disability; response to previous health care experiences; history of alcohol or drug abuse; outlook on life; and locus of control.

Sociocultural information including support systems; the age, health, and availability of significant others and their roles; family dynamics; religious influences; cultural background; social and ethnic values; health and illness beliefs of family and peers and their reactions to patient's disability; living arrangement; lifestyle; possible conflicts between culture and therapeutic recommendations.

Nursing Diagnoses: Actual or Potential

1. Altered health maintenance related to cognitive, sensory, and/ or motor deficits.
2. Self-care deficit: Feeding, bathing/hygiene, dressing/groom-

ing, toileting related to cognitive, sensory, and/or motor deficits.

3. Potential for injury related to cognitive, sensory, and/or motor deficits.
4. Impaired communication related to language and/or motor deficits.
5. Altered nutritional status: Less or more than body requirements related to swallowing deficit, inability to feed self, and/or depression.
6. Altered comfort: Pain.
7. Sleep pattern disturbances related to anxiety, pain.
8. Ineffective individual or family coping related to inadequate information, inadequate support, multiple life changes.
9. Powerlessness related to health care environment, disability related regime.
10. Disturbance in self-concept: Body image, self-esteem, role performance, personal identity.
11. Inability to access health care delivery system related to lack of knowledge and cognitive, communication, and/or motor deficits.
12. Decreased resources (financial, personal, social) for maintaining health and wellness practices.
13. Knowledge deficit regarding health and wellness management.

Expected Outcomes: Patient and/or Family

1. The individual demonstrates health maintenance practices and self-care skills appropriate to his/her developmental stage and disease/injury.
2. The individual remains free of injury.
3. The individual employs an effective method of communicating health care needs.
4. The individual maintains nutritional status as evidenced by stable body weight, normal hematocrit, hemoglobin, and serum protein.
5. The individual is comfortable as evidenced by verbal statements and/or body language.
6. The individual demonstrates an optimal balance of sleep and activity.
7. The individual experiences decreased anxiety and improved

self-concept as evidenced by verbal statements and/or body language.

8. The individual identifies community and personal resources to assist in maintaining an optimum level of health.

Planning and Implementation

The patient with cognitive impairments may not have the ability to actively participate in all aspects of wellness promotion activities. When possible use wellness teaching and behavioral strategies designed for his/her cognitive capabilities. Assist the family and/or caregivers in understanding the patient's cognitive limitations regarding health management. Assist them in learning how to provide optimal health care.

Promote positive health behaviors by reviewing with the patient and family past and current health maintenance regimes and by encouraging consistent patient involvement in developing, implementing, and evaluating wellness goals. Use appropriate methods such as behavioral programs and counseling to help the individual change high risk behaviors.

Strive to increase the perceived benefits and decrease the perceived barriers to maintaining positive health behaviors.

Provide wellness promotion activities that incorporate patients' cultural values and beliefs. Also, help them be aware of health behavior patterns in their lives and the personal meanings attached to these.

When assessing a patient's pain, be aware of the differences in pain manifestation between different cultures. For example, a stoic attitude toward pain is the accepted norm in some cultural groups while a vocal and emotional presentation is the norm in others. Awareness of these and other cultural differences in pain manifestation and presentation, plus a thorough assessment of the physiological parameters (vital signs, sleep patterns, and eating patterns) can result in a more effective pain management program. Also be aware that the pain response may be more primitive in the person with cognitive deficits and it may be more diffuse or distorted in the person with sensory deficits.

Work with the dietician to incorporate the patient's dietary preferences into meal planning instructions.

Be respectful of the patient's religious beliefs and be sensitive to

potential conflicts between the beliefs and medical recommendations.

When possible, arrange flexible visiting hours so patients, if they
desire, can have the emotional support of a more consistent family
presence.

Be aware of the patient's understanding of English and of nonverbal communication significant for his/her cultural group. If communication barriers exist, seek assistance from a person familiar with
the patient's language and culture. If a language deficit is present,
work with the speech therapist and the patient on a program to enhance communication skills. If other factors, such as a tracheostomy, interfere with communication abilities, work with the therapists and the patient to develop an alternate method of
communication.

Be respectful of the personal space preferred by the patient and
try to provide the distance or closeness that he/she is comfortable
with.

Assist the patient in learning self-care strategies to enhance wellness (nutrition, fitness, safety, positive relationship building, communication skills, and social skills).

With the patient, search for patterns and causes of stress and
anxiety and assist him/her in eliminating stressors when possible.
Facilitate further stress reduction, enhanced coping mechanisms,
increased comfort, and improved sleep patterns by teaching relaxation techniques (progressive relaxation, deep breathing, autogenic
training, guided imagery, meditation, affirmations, and self-hypno-
sis). Provide time in the patient's schedule and a soothing, supportive environment for practicing the techniques.

Use the following methods to assist the patient who has a hostile
type A personality to diffuse hostility: encourage ventilation of feelings; teach progressive relaxation exercises appropriate to the patient's physical abilities; encourage participation in recreation programs and in his/her rehabilitation program planning; and
encourage exploration of humor as a relaxation modality.

For patients who are feeling powerless and threatened by major
changes, offer them choices and participation in planning their programs to increase their sense of control. Offer them realistic challenges in a progressive manner that facilitates growth without being
overwhelming.

Facilitate patients' self-efficacy by seeking their participation in
care planning, by reinforcing their efforts at transferring their pre-

vious skills to rehabilitation, and by providing progressive learning experiences in self-care.

Use modalities such as imagery to facilitate the patient's creative problem solving abilities.

Assist the patient in reframing negative thoughts into more acceptable and helpful thoughts.

When making discharge plans with the patient, be aware of financial limitations that may affect his/her ability to follow through with health care recommendations and adjust plans accordingly.

FUTURE IMPLICATIONS

Ideally the rehabilitation experience is reflective of the wellness process. It facilitates the individual's evolution toward physical, psychological, and social integration and growth, promotes self-responsibility, awareness, motivation, and health enhancing behaviors, and it facilitates the development of coping strategies and problem solving skills. For this ideal to be achieved with each patient, further research and educational programs are needed to provide the rehabilitation nurse and other team members with more information on how psychological makeup, cultural environment, and neurological disability may affect health and wellness behaviors and on which strategies are most effective for promoting wellness in the person with a neurological disability.

REFERENCES

Ardell, D. (1985). The history and future of wellness. *Health Values, 9*:37–56.

Bandura, A. (1977). *Social learning theory.* Englewood Cliffs, NJ: Prentice Hall.

Clark, C. (1986). *Wellness nursing: Concepts, theory, research and practice.* New York: Springer Publishing Company.

Cox, C. (1985). The health self-determinism index. *Nursing Research, 34*(3):177–183.

Dembroski, T., MacDougall, J., Williams, R., Haney, T., and Blumenthal, J. (1985). Components of type A, hostility and anger in relationships to angiographic findings. *Psychosomatic Medicine, 47*(3):219–233.

Dossey, B., Keegan, L., Guzzeti, C., and Kilkneier, L. (1988). *Holistic nursing: A handbook for practice.* Rockville, MD: Aspen Publishers, Inc.

Eberst, R. (1984). Defining health: A multidimensional model. *Journal of the School of Health, 54*(3):99–104.

Frye, B. (1986). Model of wellness-seeking behavior in traumatic spinal cord injury victims. *Rehabilitation Nursing, 11*(5):6–9.

Gorton, D. (1988). Holistic health techniques to increase individual coping and wellness. *Holistic Nursing, 6*(1):25–30.

Greenberg, J. (1985). Health and wellness: A conceptual differentiation. *Journal of School Health, 55*(10):403–406.

Grimes, J., and Burns, E. (1987). *Health assessment in nursing practice* (2nd ed.). Boston: Jones and Bartlett Publishers, Inc.

Keegan, L. (1989). Discovering and actualizing the wellness potential for spinal cord injury. *SCI Nursing, 6*(1):3–7.

Keegan, L., and Dossey, B. (1987). *Self care: A program to improve your life.* Temple, TX: Bodymind Systems.

Kobasa, S., Maddi, S., and Zola, M. (1983). Type A and hardiness. *Journal of Behavioral Medicine, 6*(1):41–49.

McInerney, L. (1984). Health Education. In Howe, J., Dickason, E., Jones, D., and Snider, M. (Eds.). *The Handbook of Nursing.* New York: John Wiley and Sons.

Mumma, C. (Ed.). (1987). *Rehabilitation nursing: Concepts and practice* (2nd ed.). Evanston, IL: Rehabilitation Nursing Foundation.

Murray, R., and Zentner, J. (1985). *Nursing concepts for health promotion.* Englewood Cliffs, NJ: Prentice Hall.

Pender, N. (1982). *Health promotion in nursing practice.* Norwalk: Appleton-Century-Crofts.

Roy, C. (1984). *Introduction to nursing: An adaptation model* (2nd ed.). Englewood Cliffs, NJ: Prentice Hall.

Shaver, J. (1985). A biopsychosocial view of health. *Nursing Outlook, 33*(4):186–191.

Siegel, J. (1984). Type A behavior: Epidemiologic foundations and public health implications. *Annual Review of Public Health, 5*:343–367.

Stephens, P. (1987). Experience of health and illness. In Lewis, S., and Collier, I. (Eds.). *Medical surgical nursing: Assessment and management of clinical problems.* New York: McGraw Hill Book Company.

Patient and Family Education

2

OBJECTIVES

After completing this chapter, the reader will be able to:

- Discuss the differences between learning and teaching.
- Describe the neurophysiological basis of learning.
- Discuss the three domains of learning and the abilities associated with each domain.
- Discuss learner characteristics and explain how each may affect the individual's motivation and ability to learn.
- Review the characteristics that can affect the nurse's effectiveness as a teacher.
- Discuss teaching interventions and the special considerations needed for the cognitively impaired patient.
- Describe methods for evaluating learning.

INTRODUCTION

For persons with neurological disabilities to achieve and maintain a high level of wellness they must have access to a multidimensional education program. This program must address the physical, cognitive, psychological, and sociocultural dimensions of their lives and offer opportunities for them to learn new skills and adaptive behaviors. Because of the tremendous variations in neurological status, abilities, and life circumstances, teaching plans must be individualized to meet the unique needs of each person.

The rehabilitation nurse has an integral role in all aspects of patient education. Primary responsibilities within the role include facilitating learning through the use of appropriate teaching and rehabilitation methodologies and providing a caring environment that is supportive of each patient's personal exploration and growth.

DEFINITIONS OF LEARNING AND TEACHING

Learning is the acquisition of knowledge, attitudes, and skills that lead to behavioral changes. It is a dynamic multidimensional process influenced by a person's previous life experiences and current psychological and physical status. Learning is motivated by the individual's attempt to resolve unmet problems or needs. Memory and learning are closely related, as memory is the process whereby learned information is stored in the central nervous system for future retrieval.

Teaching is the plan of action that is designed to bring about learning or that allows it to occur. The process of teaching has the same basic components as the nursing process. An assessment is made of the patient's and family's learning needs, motivation, and ability to learn. Following the assessment, learning objectives are established. A teaching plan is then developed based on the assessment data and learning objectives. After implementation of the teaching plan, its effectiveness is determined by evaluating whether the adaptive behaviors have been achieved.

NEUROPHYSIOLOGICAL BASIS OF LEARNING

Memory is the primary cognitive process associated with learning, though any number of cognitive processes may be involved, depending on the nature of the learning activities. Memory is thought to involve the encoding, storage, and retrieval of information, though these components are difficult to separate. Encoding refers to the process by which a memory of physical objects and events is developed. Storage refers to the persistence of the information over time. Retrieval refers to the search for and utilization of stored information.

There are two separate memory systems: procedural memory is knowing how to perform an activity, declarative memory is memory for facts and information. There is no neural pathway which directly connects the two systems, but they may share physiological mechanisms.

Procedural memory is acquired through repetitive activity and manifested in performance of a skill or habit. The response is stored in the memory system, not information about the response. This process involves interaction between the motor cortex and the subcortical motor areas including the basal ganglia. Procedural memory is more diffuse than declarative memory and is activated on an unconscious level.

Declarative memory is acquired by receiving and recognizing sensory stimuli through watching, listening, or having tactile experiences. It is mediated through the corticolimbic system. It must be consciously activated, but does not require multiple repetitions for storage. There are three subsystems of declarative memory: immediate, short-term, and long-term memories.

Immediate memory (working memory) is memory of a few numbers, words, phrases, or other bits of information after a few seconds. It has a very limited storage capacity and is distraction labile, meaning a new stimulus cannot be introduced while a memory is being held in the immediate memory store or that memory will be lost. Impairment in this system is manifested as inattentiveness, distractibility, or failure to focus on the stimulus.

Short-term memory (recent memory) is memory of a few numbers, words, letters, phrases, or other bits of information after a few minutes. Short-term memory stores are distraction stable compared to immediate memory stores, enabling the individual to attend to other stimuli without losing the memory held in the short-term memory system. Impairment in this system is manifested as an anterograde amnesia.

For a short-term memory to be retained it must be transferred to long-term memory stores. A long-term memory (remote, permanent, or fixed memory) is the memory of information that can be recalled minutes or years later. It is stored primarily in the cortical association areas. Impairment in this system is manifested as a retrograde amnesia. Each hemisphere processes and stores long-term memories differently. The left hemisphere uses sequential analysis to process and store component parts of memories related to language, math calculations, and abstractions. The right hemisphere uses a holistic method to process and store memories involving visual experiences, spatial relationships, and non-language sounds such as music.

For long-term memories to be retrieved later, the neural pathway must become permanent through a process called consolidation (encoding and storage). The limbic system, especially the hippocampus, amygdala, and adjacent areas of the temporal lobe, are involved in the transfer, consolidation, and retrieval processes. Anatomical and chemical changes in the neurons also appear to be involved. Reprocessing of memories by the prefrontal areas leads to an increase in the depth and abstractness of different thoughts (elaboration of thought). Brain injury or disease that damages the cortical association areas, prefrontal areas, temporal lobe, and/or parts of the limbic system can disrupt any of the components of memory encoding, storage, retrieval, and reprocessing. Destruction of cortical tissue can destroy memory stores.

DOMAINS OF LEARNING

Learning is classified into three domains: cognitive, psychomotor, and affective. In developing a teaching plan the nurse must identify the domain in which learning is to occur, whether impairment exists in that domain, and the appropriate teaching and compensatory strategies related to that domain. The cognitive domain, as it is usually addressed, involves primarily left hemisphere learning: fact (memorization) and concept (classification or categorization) learning taught through verbal presentations and written information, and problem solving (application of facts and concepts to other situations) taught through discussion. With successful cognitive learning (involving long-term declarative memory system and thought elaboration) the learner in the rehabilitation setting is able to recall factual information regarding health and disability management to interpret and synthesize this information, to apply the concepts to real life situations, to compare relationships of different concepts, to synthesize the information and form hypotheses, and to problem solve and make judgments.

As discussed previously, the person with brain damage may have mild to severe difficulties with declarative memory and cognitive learning. Therefore modifications will need to be made in the teaching plan to address his/her specific needs. For example, persons with declarative memory system impairments can be helped to acquire learned responses to stimulus situations such as eating and dressing. This is accomplished with a structured program involving consistent stimuli and feedback designed to elicit and maintain the desired response. Persons with procedural memory system impairments may be retrained in a skill by reestablishing a pathway through repetition or by substituting one skill for another. Informational learning in their declarative memory systems can be enhanced by reducing or clearly defining nonessential information and by encouraging rehearsal and integration of new information. It is also essential that family members and/or caregivers are involved in all stages of the teaching learning process.

Learning in the psychomotor domain concerns the individual's ability to perform skilled physical activities within the limitations of his/her neuromuscular deficits. The right and left hemispheres are involved in psychomotor learning in the following ways: the right incorporates the visual and spatial concepts (right declarative memory system) and the left incorporates the verbal instructions and the sequencing of the activities (procedural memory system). With successful psychomotor learning the learner develops skill in following directions and carrying out activities according to these directions. He/she demonstrates improved coordination and over time is able to carry out activities without a model or instructions. He/she is able to coordinate multiple activities by establishing an appropriate sequence and is ultimately able to perform an activity in an almost automatic way.

The affective domain involves changing attitudes and behavior and combines elements of both declarative and procedural memory and right and left hemisphere activities. Activity within this domain strongly impacts on whether individuals are able to successfully adapt to their disabilities. Affective learning is taught through role modeling, role playing, and group discussion. With successful affective learning the learner develops greater self awareness and assumes more personal responsibility. He/she is able to conceptualize personal values and is willing to consider alternatives and change opinions in light of new information.

LEARNER CHARACTERISTICS AND FACTORS AFFECTING MOTIVATION AND ABILITY TO LEARN

Neurological Status

As discussed previously, a person who has incurred damage to the cortical association areas, temporal lobes, limbic system, and/or the prefrontal association areas through trauma or disease will have some degree of learning dysfunction due to memory impairment and attention deficits. In such a situation one memory system may be damaged and the other left intact, or both may be damaged, depending on the location and extent of the trauma or disease. Hemispheric damage will affect how an individual is able to store and retrieve information. A person with right hemisphere damage is most likely to have difficulty with verbal learning, math calculations, and abstractions. The person with left hemisphere damage is most likely to have difficulty with visual and perceptual learning. Other types of disease or trauma-related cognitive impairments can also affect a person's learning ability. These include language disturbances and impaired abstract thinking, generalization, problem solving, and executive function.

Motor deficits and spatial perceptual problems can interfere with psychomotor learning. Pain can adversely affect the individual's motivation and ability to concentrate and attend to learning activities. Sensory deficits such as visual and hearing impairments will affect the type of teaching methods that can be used.

Developmental Level

The adolescent learner tends to be egocentric and self absorbed. Striving for peer approval, privacy, and independence are major developmental concerns. After sustaining a disability, the ability to resolve these concerns may be seriously compromised.

The young and middle aged adult learner desires immediacy of application of teaching, needs to integrate new ideas into established patterns, may have some limited knowledge of learning materials but this may be distorted by misconceptions, is reality and problem oriented, and is concerned about preserving self-esteem.

With the aged learner, maintaining independence is a prime learning motivator. Imprinting new learning requires more time and the use of association and previous learning. Sensory impairments may interfere with learning. Information tends to be processed better visually rather than auditorially. Other characteristics include physical limitations (in addition to disability-related limitations) of decreased strength, endurance, and speed; impaired perceptual ability with decreased vision and hearing; and egocentricity with well-established patterns.

Gender

Females tend to have increased hearing acuity and a larger vocabulary, use bilateral hemispheres, and are better at fine motor skills. Males tend to have visual superiority, use the right hemisphere more, and have better coordination with gross motor skills.

Locus of Control

A person with an internal locus of control tends to feel in control of life's events, copes better with threatening situations, and perceives the relationship between behavior and the results. He/she tends to be focused on long-term gains and is more willing to forego immediate rewards to achieve these. He/she usually responds well to health promotion and independent study programs.

A person with an external locus of control tends to feel helpless and powerless in the face of problems. These feelings of helplessness and powerlessness are further reinforced after the individual has sustained a disability. He/she usually responds best to structured group programs. Being from a lower socioeconomic or minority group may contribute to the development of an external viewpoint.

In addition to neurological status, developmental level, and locus of control, the patient's level of fatigue, anxiety, depression, fear, denial, and anger can all affect his/her motivation and ability to learn. Conflicts associated with health and cultural beliefs and values, interpersonal influences, time constraints, financial problems, and the complexity of the management plan can also adversely affect the patient's motivation and ability to learn.

Maslow's needs theory and Rosenstock's Health Belief Model provide additional insights into the factors that affect motivation and learning ability (in the person with no or minimal cognitive impairment). In Maslow's theory, motivation is defined as the process by which behavior is initiated in response to a need (Mumma, 1987).

People experiencing an illness or disability often find themselves in situations where they need assistance to manage their most basic needs such as eating and elimination (Maslow's Level 1—physiological and survival needs). According to this theory, needs are hierarchical and interdependent with deficits on one level affecting other levels. Therefore, being forced to return to a basic need level will greatly affect the person's motivation and ability to address higher order needs (the higher level needs are, in ascending order: Level 2—safety and security, 3—love, affection, and belongingness, 4—esteem, 5—self-actualization).

In Rosenstock's model (Mumma, 1987) motivation and ability to learn are affected by the following: the individual's perception of the probability of experiencing illness or complications, the individual's perception of the severity of the potential illness and the impact on his/her life, the perceived benefits of preventive action, and the cost of health action in money, time, effort, and side effects.

NURSE TEACHER CHARACTERISTICS

Many factors can affect the nurse's effectiveness as a teacher. Therefore, he/she needs to perform an ongoing self-assessment in order to identify personal strengths and deficits in the area of patient teaching and to create a self-development program that will enhance the strengths and overcome the deficits. Peer evaluation, audio- and video-taping of teaching sessions, as well as learner feedback, can provide additional information for a more complete self-assessment. The following list presents some of the attributes of an effective nurse teacher.

Adequate knowledge of the subjects to be taught and the available resources.

Knowledge of theories of learning neurophysiology, related pathophysiology, and knowledge of teaching techniques that will maximize learning.

Communication skills to adapt communication methods for each patient's comprehension ability.

Interpersonal skills to provide the ability to listen and create a climate of trust that puts patients and families at ease, and the ability to convey interest and respect that facilitates active involvement in the education program.

Time management skills to structure responsibilities so that teaching time is integrated into the daily plans.

Positive attitudes about the patient, teaching, and the subjects to be taught; awareness of the importance of nonverbal as well as verbal communication to convey acceptance, respect, and interest.

NURSING INTERVENTIONS

To develop an effective patient and family education program the nurse must obtain pertinent information regarding the learner's demographic, cognitive, physical, psychological, and sociocultural status. The planning and implementation process should then become an integration of this information, the identified learning needs, and the appropriate subject content and teaching methodologies.

Learner Assessment

Demographic information including age, marital status, occupation, education level, ability to read and write, primary language, and financial status.

Cognitive information including brain disease or injury related impairments (attention deficits, memory deficits, impaired abstraction, generalization, concept formation, and problem solving abilities, language disturbances, and executive deficits); learning style, level of intelligence, history of learning disability, perceived information needs and priorities, current level of knowledge about disability, health expectations, and past experiences that may prepare for present learning.

Physical information including musculoskeletal limitations, diminished visual and hearing acuity, reduced tolerance secondary to pain, fatigue, and/or deconditioning.

Psychological information including presence of affective disorders related to brain damage, presence of fear, anxiety, and depression; type and effectiveness of coping style; level of maturity; self image; personal meaning of disability; response to previous health care experiences; history of alcohol or drug abuse; outlook on life; locus of control.

Sociocultural information including support systems; age, health, and availability of significant others and their roles; family dynamics; religious influences; cultural background; social and ethnic values; attitudes and beliefs of family and peers and their reactions to patient's disability; living arrangement; lifestyle; possible conflicts between culture and therapeutic recommendations.

Planning and Implementation

Determine if the patient is a candidate for learning based on the assessment findings. if conditions such as pain, fatigue, or anxiety interfere with the individual's learning readiness, work with him/her to reduce or eliminate the problem. If cognitive deficits limit the individual's ability to learn, include the family or other care givers in all teaching interventions.

With the patient and/or family establish realistic learning goals and objectives and measurable time-related outcomes. Goal achievement is more likely when these goals are related to the self-identified needs of the learner. Also realistic, attainable goals provide mechanisms for feedback, which motivates further learning.

Select the subject content that fulfills the learning objectives and is appropriate to the learner's cognitive, physical, and psychological capabilities. Determine the number of sessions required by breaking the content down into meaningful parts.

Prioritize information or practice based on the immediacy of the learning need. The need is acute if the patient will be in physical or emotional danger without the information or response. Preventive needs apply to information or responses that are needed to eliminate or decrease the possibility of illness or complications. Maintenance needs relate to self-care information and activities.

Organize the content presentation or practice from simple to complex. For declarative information organize from concrete to abstract. Begin with what the learner knows and build on this.

Select teaching strategies appropriate to the learner's learning style, locus of control, developmental level, and gender (discussion/lecture, verbal presentation/demonstration, group/individual instruction/independent study).

Pace learning activities according to the learner's physical tolerance and cognitive abilities.

Select instructional materials to supplement the teaching methodology based on the learner's cognitive, visual, and hearing abilities, learning style, verbal/reading comprehension. Provide opportunities for follow-up discussion when audiovisual or printed materials are used.

Consider the nature of learning required (whether the declarative or procedural memory system will be used) and the related learning domain. Select teaching strategies related to that memory system and learning domain.

Cognitive domain/declarative memory system:

- To maximize informational learning, reduce distractions and the amount of other nonessential information received by the immediate and short-term memory subsystems.
- Associate new learning with old.
- Encourage rehearsals of new information by creating learning situations where the learner is able to reuse the information to form new associations.
- Assist the learner to see the relationship between specific facts, principles, and generalizations.

Select teaching strategies that will maximize the abilities and minimize the deficits of the cognitively impaired patient.

For attention, memory, and integration problems in general:

- Provide a non-threatening, predictable, distraction-free environment.
- Maintain consistency and structure in scheduling and in learning activities.
- Provide simple instructions that are repeated throughout the session.
- Use memory aids as needed.
- Allow adequate time for responses.
- Keep sessions brief.

For impaired left hemisphere and intact right hemisphere function:

- Use visual and spatial teaching methods and flexible progression of content.
- Use behavioral techniques (procedural memory) that provide consistent stimuli and feedback.

For impaired right hemisphere and intact left hemisphere function:

- Provide sequential progression of teaching via verbal and written methods.
- Use behavioral techniques (procedural memory) that provide consistent stimuli and feedback.

Provide family members of the cognitively impaired patient with information to help them understand the nature of the problem and the pathophysiological reasons for the patient's behavior. Assist them in learning how to work with the patient to maximize abilities, minimize disability-related limitations, and prevent complications.

Provide a physically comfortable learning environment that is temperature controlled, well lit, easily accessible, and free of visual and auditory distractions.

Convey attitudes that will enhance learning: value the material being taught, convey interest in teaching, and demonstrate acceptance of the learner.

Provide ongoing feedback to facilitate learning, promote self confidence, and further motivate the learner.

EVALUATION

Evaluating learning involves comparing the expected learning outcomes with the learner's actual behavior following teaching. Evaluations are also used to judge the effectiveness of the teaching and the appropriateness of the teaching materials.

The method by which any evaluation is conducted depends on the domain of learning that is used. With the topic cognitive domain, learning outcomes are stated in terms of knowledge the learner will acquire. With the affective domain, outcomes are stated in terms of what the learner will become or what will characterize the learner as development takes place. With the psychomotor domain, outcomes will be specified as measurable behaviors or performance.

A learner centered approach to evaluation includes activities such as informing the learner of when the evaluation will take place and the type of questions to be asked. This type of evaluation is also structured to focus on the learner's successes in an effort to promote self responsibility.

An ongoing or formative evaluation facilitates planning adjustments based on the learner's current needs and provides the learner with feedback so that desirable behavior can be reinforced and undesirable behavior redirected. Data for this type of evaluation is gained primarily from questions, responses, and nonverbal behavior.

A summative evaluation determines how well the learner has learned after teaching is completed and whether any unexpected outcomes occurred as a result of the teaching process. This evaluation conveys information about the effectiveness of the entire teaching process while the formative evaluation conveys information about how things are going during the teaching process. Data for the summative evaluation is gained from written and oral tests, checklists, rating scales, and performance observations.

When giving feedback to the learner during or following the evaluation, the nurse should initially provide positive reinforcement for the desired behavior before discussing areas that still need improvement. Absolutes like "always" and "never" should be avoided. When information is shared, alternatives should be presented so the learner can make some independent decisions. When specific suggestions are offered, the rationale for each should be given. Feedback should be given as soon as possible after the evaluation. When providing feedback to the patient with brain damage use feedback mechanisms that he/she is most responsive to in light of the specific cognitive impairments.

In addition to the evaluation of the learner, the teaching program and the nurse's role must also be evaluated to facilitate future program planning and presentations. The following questions address this broader evaluation dimension:

- Were the goals mutually agreed upon, realistic, and timely?
- Were educational needs adequately identified and defined?
- Were the results of the learner assessment taken into consideration when developing the teaching plan?
- Was the learner's self respect and sense of control maintained?
- Was positive feedback given on an ongoing basis?

FUTURE IMPLICATIONS

For an education program to be effective, information must be directed not only to the patient's understanding of his/her disability and treatment but also toward the adaptation and behavioral changes that will produce optimum wellness. To facilitate these changes the rehabilitation nurse must have an understanding of all the dimensions of the individual's life, how these impact on learning, and how to successfully incorporate this information into the teaching plan.

Research and education programs are providing rehabilitation nurses and other members of the health care community with information on how psychosocial and cultural variables affect learning and on how to develop learning assessment and teaching methodologies that address these variables. In addition, research programs that are investigating the mechanisms involved in memory and learning are providing new insights and information on methods to assess and facilitate learning in persons with brain damage and other neurological disabilities.

However, in spite of progress in these areas, in most facilities chronic problems exist that interfere with the nurse's ability to consistently provide effective patient education. Overcoming these problems of limited time for teaching interventions, limited funds for obtaining teaching tools, and limited opportunities for participating in professional education programs remains an ongoing challenge. While individual institutions may be able to meet this challenge on a short-term basis, long-term universal solutions will not be found until underlying problems such as the nursing shortage and escalating health care costs have been successfully addressed on a national level.

REFERENCES

Blattner, B. (1986). *Holistic nursing.* Englewood Cliffs: Prentice Hall, Inc.

Boss, B. (1985). New neuroanatomical and neurophysiological basis of learning. *Journal of Neuroscience Nursing, 18*(5):256–264.

Bower, G., and Hilgard, E. (1981). *Theories of learning* (5th ed.). Englewood Cliffs: Prentice Hall, Inc.

Cahill, M. (Ed.). (1987). *Patient teaching.* Springhouse: Springhouse Corporation.

Collins, C. (1989). Perceived learning needs for rehabilitation following spinal cord injury. *SCI Nursing, 6*(1):8–13.

Falvo, D. (1985). *Effective patient education: A guide to increased compliance.* Rockville: Aspen System Corporation.

Ford, R. (Ed.). (1987). *Patient teaching manual 1 and 2.* Springhouse: Springhouse Corporation.

Hanak, M. (Ed.). (1990). *Education guide for spinal cord injury nurses: A manual for teaching patients, families, and caregivers.* New York: American Association of Spinal Cord Injury Nurses.

Hanak, M. (1986). *Patient and family education: Teaching programs for managing chronic diseases and disability.* New York: Springer Publishing Company.

Mumma, C. (Ed.). (1987). *Rehabilitation nursing: Concepts and practice* (2nd ed.). Evanston: Rehabilitation Nursing Foundation.

Nielson, L. (1989). Client and family learning in the rehabilitation setting. *Nursing Clinics of North America, 24*:257–264.

Stull, P. (1985). *Effective teaching tips.* Baltimore: Resource Applications, Incorporated.

Stull, P. (1985). *Improve your instructional skills.* Baltimore: Resource Applications, Incorporated.

Ward, D. (1986). Why patient teaching fails. *Rehabilitation Nursing, 49*(1):45–47.

Waters, J. (1987). Learning needs of spinal cord injured patients. *Rehabilitation Nursing, 12*(6):309–312.

Neuroanatomy and Physiology Review

3

OBJECTIVES

After completing this chapter, the reader will be able to:

- Identify the primary protective structures surrounding the brain.
- Discuss the mechanisms involved in cerebral circulation. Identify the primary cerebral arteries and the areas of the brain they supply.
- Identify the structures of the cerebrum. Describe the functions associated with each structure and the impairments resulting from damage to these structures.
- Identify the structures and functions of the diencephalon and the brain stem. Explain the relationship between the brain stem and the reticular formation.
- Identify the cranial nerves. Describe the associated functions and the impairments resulting from damage to each nerve.
- Outline the divisions of the vertebral column, noting the number of vertebrae in each division.
- Identify the spinal cord tracts and the associated functions.
- Describe the structure of the spinal nerves and their role in reflex activities.
- Describe the functions associated with each division of the autonomic nervous system.

INTRODUCTION

Because of the integrated relationship between the divisions of the nervous system (central, peripheral, and autonomic) persons with neurological disabilities are likely to have some degree of functional impairment in each of these divisions. Thus the ways in which they receive sensory information, process and store this information, and generate voluntary and involuntary motor impulses may all be affected.

Knowledge of neuroanatomy and pathophysiology enables the rehabilitation nurse to more fully understand the functional changes experienced by persons with neurological disabilities and the possible psychological and sociocultural effects of these changes. He/she can then provide the appropriate intervention that will assist these individuals in moving toward reintegration and wellness.

BRAIN ANATOMY AND PHYSIOLOGY

Cranium, Meninges, and Cerebrospinal Fluid (CSF)

The cranium is the part of the skull that encloses the brain. It is composed of the frontal, occipital, sphenoid, ethmoid, parietal, and temporal bones. These bones are joined by four major sutures: the sagittal suture joining the parietal bones, the coronal (frontoparietal) suture, the lambdoid (occipitoparietal) suture, and the basal suture joining the basilar surface of the occipital bone with the posterior surface of the sphenoid bone.

The brain is covered by three protective meninges. The outermost double meningeal layer is the dura mater. The subdural space separates the dura from the middle meningeal layer, the arachnoid. The subarachnoid space is between the arachnoid and the innermost meningeal layer, the pia mater. The subarachnoid space and the ventricles of the brain contain cerebrospinal fluid (CSF), a clear, colorless solution that acts as a shock absorber to cushion the brain. It is formed primarily in the choroid plexus located in portions of the lateral, third, and fourth ventricles. The CSF is reabsorbed through the arachnoid villi into the venous sinuses of the brain at an average rate of 500cc daily.

Cerebral Circulation

The cerebral blood flow (CBF) accounts for approximately 17% of the cardiac output. It transports 20% of the body's oxygen supply to the brain for the oxidation of glucose. The brain is totally dependent on this oxidation process for its metabolism. A 2- to 5-minute lack of oxygen can result in irreversible brain damage. Four intrinsic regulatory mechanisms assure a constant blood flow to the brain: cerebral autoregulation, cerebral perfusion pressure, carbon dioxide level, and cerebrovascular resistance. Extrinsic influencing factors include blood pressure, blood viscosity, and head position. A barrier system, composed of the blood brain barrier, the blood CSF barrier, and the brain CSF barrier, regulates the transport of nutrients, ions, water, and waste products between the plasma, CSF, and the brain. The barrier system influences brain function by determining the level of metabolism and ionic composition.

Table 3-1 identifies the primary cerebral arteries and the areas of the brain they supply. The veins of the cerebral circulation drain into the superior longitudinal sinus, the cavernosus sinus, and the

TABLE 3-1 Primary Cerebral Arteries

I. Internal carotid
   *A. Anterior cerebral—supplies medial surface of frontal and parietal lobes
   *B. Middle Cerebral—supplies lateral surface of frontal, parietal, temporal, and occipital lobes
   C. Ophthalmic—supplies orbits
   D. Anterior choroidal—supplies choroid plexus
   *E. Posterior communicating—joins posterior cerebral and internal carotids
   *F. Anterior communicating—joins anterior cerebrals
II. Vertebrobasilar
   A. Anterior inferior cerebellar, posterior inferior cerebellar, superior cerebellar, and inferior cerebellar—supply cerebellum
   B. Bulbar—supplies medulla
   C. Pontine—supplies pons
   *D. Posterior cerebral—supplies inferior and medial surface of temporal and occipital lobes and parts of diencephalon, midbrain, and optic pathway

*The Circle of Willis forms an anastomosis between the internal carotids and vertebrobasilar system providing a means of collateral circulation. It is the origin of the anterior, middle, and posterior cerebral arteries.

inferior longitudinal sinus. These sinuses empty into the dural sinus which in turn empties into the jugular veins which return the blood to the heart.

Cerebrum (Telencephalon)

The brain is divided into three main areas: the cerebrum, the brain stem, and the cerebellum. The cerebrum is the largest area, accounting for 4/5 of the total brain weight. It is composed of the cerebral hemispheres, thalamus, hypothalamus, and basal ganglia. The two hemispheres are separated by the great longitudinal fissure and connected at the base by the corpus callosum. The outer layer of the cerebrum is covered by the cortex. Each hemisphere is divided into four lobes using the major folds of the cortex as landmarks (Figure 3-1). The central fissure of Rolando separates the frontal from the parietal lobes and separates the anterior and posterior areas of each hemisphere. The lateral fissure of Sylvius separates the temporal from the frontal and parietal lobes. The parieto-occipital fissure separates the occipital lobe from the parietal and temporal lobes.

Functional mapping of the brain has been attempted through the

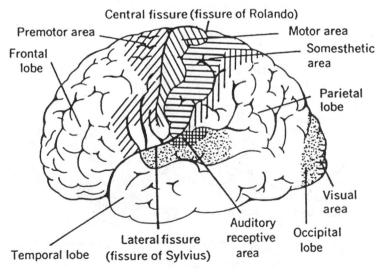

FIGURE 3-1 Lobes and functional areas of cerebral hemisphere. (Hickey, J: *The Clinical Practice of Neurological and Neurosurgical Nursing* [2nd ed.] Philadelphia: J. B. Lippincott Co., 1986.)

study of the effects of brain damage, electrical stimulation, neuro-surgical procedures, and neuroanatomical studies coupled with animal research. As a result the brain is now thought to be organized in both a focal and a diffuse manner. Primary sensory and motor functions are controlled by specific regions in each lobe called primary areas. The integration of higher level functions occurs in the association areas of each lobe.

Frontal Lobes

Within the frontal lobes are the primary motor areas which direct voluntary control over movement. These primary areas are topologically arranged so there is a systematic, orderly representation in the cortex of different parts of the body (Figure 3-2). Each cortical region projects to specific muscles in the opposite side of the body. The premotor areas are involved with higher level motor organization. Damage to the primary motor areas results in paralysis while damage to the premotor areas results in disturbance in or-

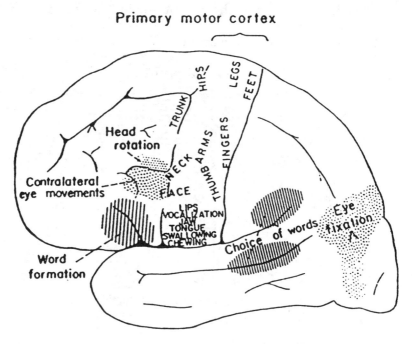

FIGURE 3-2 Primary motor areas. (Guyton, A: *Structure and Function of the Nervous System* [2nd ed.] Philadelphia: W. B. Saunders, 1976.)

ganization of movement. Broca's area lies at the inferior frontal gyrus and controls the expressive aspects of language. Lesions in this area result in expressive aphasia. The remaining portions of the frontal lobes are called the prefrontal areas. These areas are involved with higher integrative functions such as attention, concentration, memory, abstraction generalization, problem solving, and executive function, judgment, and the mediation of personality. Damage results in both cognitive and personality changes.

Parietal Lobes

The somesthetic or primary sensory areas are located in the post central gyrus at the parietal lobes. These areas represent the termination of the pathways dealing with general sensations of touch, pressure, pain, heat and cold, and joint and limb position. They provide information about the localization of the sensory stimulus but not about the quality. Information concerning the quality of the stimulus (differences in intensity, textural differences, and spatial discrimination) is provided by the sensory association areas. Connections between the primary sensory areas, the sensory association areas, and the visual and auditory areas permit an interrelationship of several sensory inputs (Figure 3-3). Damage to the

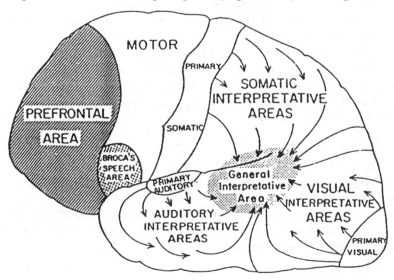

FIGURE 3-3 Sensory association areas. (Guyton, A: *Structure and Function of the Nervous System* [2nd ed.] Philadelphia, W. B. Saunders, 1976.)

primary sensory association areas results in a variety of sensory-perceptual impairments such as agnosia, anosognosia, astereognosia, hyperalgesia, and hyperesthesia.

Occipital Lobes

The primary visual receptive areas occupy a large part of the occipital lobes. Input to these areas is provided by fibers originating in the retina. The visual association areas provide interpretation of visual experiences. Damage to these areas results in visual agnosia cortical blindness, and altitudinal and depth misperceptions.

Temporal Lobes

The temporal lobes contain the primary auditory areas which translate nerve impulses into sounds. The auditory association areas interpret auditory experiences and provide auditory memory storage. Damage to these areas results in auditory agnosia. Wernicke's area, located in the dominant temporal and inferior parietal lobe, is involved with expressive language. Damage to this area results in expressive aphasia. The hippocampus, located in the medial portion of the temporal lobe, plays a critical role in memory system function. Hippocampal damage results in the inability to transfer items from short-term to long-term memory. The interpretive area is located in the supramarginal and angular gyri of the temporal lobe (where the temporal, parietal, and occipital lobes meet). This area provides an integration of the visual, auditory, and somatic areas and is involved in memory storage. Damage to this area in the dominant temporal lobe usually results in severe impairment of intellectual ability. The temporal lobes are also involved in olfactory perception.

Myelinated Fibers

The myelinated fibers (white matter) of the cerebrum include the projection fibers, which connect the cortex with the subcortical structures and the spinal cord, the association fibers, which connect adjacent or distinct gyri in the same hemisphere, and the commissural fibers (corpus callosum), which connect corresponding regions of the two hemispheres.

Basal Ganglia

The basal ganglia are large masses of gray matter located deep in the cerebral hemispheres. They include the caudate nucleus, lenticular nucleus (globus pallidus and putamen), amygdaloid nucleus, and the claustrum. The caudate and lenticular nuclei constitute the corpus striatum. The role of the basal ganglia in conjunction with the substantia nigra, subthalamic nuclei, and the dentate nucleus is to facilitate fine motor control and postural movements and to suppress certain types of motor function that would destroy the purposeful nature of the motor activity. Damage to these structures results in dysfunctional movements such as the muscle rigidity, tremor and bradykinesia seen in Parkinson's disease.

Diencephalon

The thalamus constitutes about 80% of the diencephalon. It functions as a sensory relay station between the cerebellum and the cerebrum. It also provides a crude translation of sensory input as pleasant or unpleasant. Lesions within the sensory portions of the thalamus result in a thalamic syndrome characterized by nonspecific, spontaneous, and excruciating pain.

Output from the phytothalamus travels via nerves or chemicals to the pituitary gland, the limbic system, and the midbrain and from there to the body viscera. The primary functions of the hypothalamus are concerned with the regulation of homeostatic functions (autonomic activities, temperature regulation, food intake, water metabolism, pituitary function, sleep-wakefulness, and libido). Connection between the hypothalamus, cingulate gyrus, and the temporal lobes are considered an anatomic unit called the limbic system. This system does not represent an actual area of the brain but rather identifies the interrelationship of these areas in the expression of emotion and visceral function. Damage results in behavioral and visceral function changes.

The brain stem is composed of the midbrain, pons, medulla, and the reticular formation. The midbrain carries motor projection fibers from the cerebrum to the spinal cord and the cerebellum. It contains neuron cell bodies that give rise to the tectospinal and rubrospinal tracts. It also contains the substantia nigra. The nuclei of oculomotor (III) and the trochlea (IV) cranial nerves are located here. Midbrain lesions typically affect visual movement and produce deficits in voluntary movement such as decerebrate posturing.

The pons consist of fibers descending to the spinal cord (corticospinal fibers) and from the pons to the cerebellum (pontocerebellar fibers). It contains nuclei of the trigeminal (V), abducent (VI), facial

(VII), and vestibulocochlear (VIII) cranial nerves. The pneumotaxic center is also located in the pons. Damage to the pons results in motor deficits, facial sensory and motor impairments, hearing and balance problems, and impaired breathing.

The vital centers are located within the medulla. The cardiac center sends impulses to regulate heart rate according to the body's activity level and need for oxygen. The respiratory center regulates inspiration and exhalation and the vasomotor centers control blood pressure. Nonvital centers involved with swallowing, vomiting, sneezing, and coughing are also located in the medulla. Integrated with the functions of the vital and nonvital centers are the nuclei of the glossopharyngeal (IX), vagus (X), accessory (XI), and hypoglossal (XII) cranial nerves. Corticospinal fibers cross over in the medulla and ascending sensory fibers synapse here. Damage to the medulla results in vasomotor and respiratory dysfunction, uncontrolled vomiting, and motor and sensory deficits.

The reticular formation receives input from most of the sensory systems of the body and from the cerebral motor region. Damage to this area results in arousal, attention, immediate memory system, and perceptual deficits. The upper part of the formation plus the pathways to the thalamus and cortex are called the reticular activating system (RAS), which aids in maintaining the conscious state. A coma is indicative of RAS damage.

Cerebellum

The cerebellum is composed of the cerebellar cortex, the white matter which forms connecting pathways for afferent and efferent impulses joining the cerebellum with other parts of the CNS, and four cerebellar nuclei. The primary functions of the cerebellum are to insure that movement goes where it is supposed to at the proper rate and force, to insure smooth movements, to calculate when a motion should be slowed and stopped, and to insure that muscle groups contract in a particular order. Manifestations of cerebellar dysfunction include asthenia, greater fatigue of muscles on the side of the damage, loss of muscle tone, ataxia, and balance problems.

Cranial Nerves

The peripheral nervous system is composed of the cranial nerves and the spinal nerves. Table 3-2 identifies the cranial nerves and their primary functions.

TABLE 3-2 Cranial Nerves and Their Primary Functions

Nerve	Function
I. Olfactory (sensory)	Smell
II. Optic (sensory)	Vision
III. Oculomotor (motor)	Pupil constriction and accommodation, extraocular movement
IV. Trochlear (motor)	Downward and inward eye movement
V. Trigeminal (motor, sensory)	Chewing, sensation in front of head, sneezing reflex
VI. Abducens (motor)	Lateral eye movement
VII. Facial (motor, sensory)	Face movements, salivation, crying, taste
VIII. Acoustic (sensory)	Hearing, balance
IX. Glossopharyngeal (motor, sensory)	Swallowing, salivation, taste
X. Vagus (motor, sensory, autonomic)	Swallowing, taste, vocalization, autonomic innervation
XI. Spinal accessory (motor)	Turning head, lifting shoulders
XII. Hypoglossal (motor)	Tongue movement

SPINAL CORD ANATOMY AND PHYSIOLOGY

The vertebral column protects the spinal cord, supports the head, and provides flexibility. It is composed of seven cervical vertebrae (C1-7), 12 thoracic vertebrae (T1-12), five lumbar vertebrae (L1-5), five fused sacral vertebrae (S1-5), and four fused coccygeal vertebrae (Figure 3-4). The typical vertebra has an anterior portion, the vertebral body, a posterior portion, the neural arch, and transverse, spinous, and articular processes. The spinal cord runs through the vertebral canal which is formed by the junction of the vertebral body and the neural arch. The supporting structures that give the spine stability include the anterior and posterior longitudinal ligaments, the intervertebral disks, and the trunk and neck musculature.

Spinal Cord

The spinal cord extends from the medulla oblongata just above the foramen magnum to the upper border of the second lumbar vertebra where it comes to a tapered end called the conus medullaris.

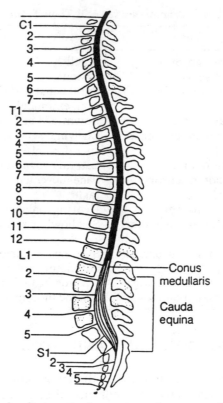

FIGURE 3-4 Vertebral column. (Buchanan, L., and Nawoczenski, D: *Spinal Cord Injury: Concepts and Management Approaches.* Baltimore, Williams and Wilkins, 1987.)

Nerve roots extending down the spinal canal from this point are called the cauda equina. The spinal cord is surrounded by the three protective meninges. Cerebrospinal fluid (CSF) is contained within the space separating the arachnoid from the pia mater. A central canal containing CSF runs through the cord from the fourth ventricle in the medulla oblongata to the end of the conus medullaris. The arterial blood supply to the cord is carried by the anterior and two posterior arteries, which arise from the vertebral arteries at the foramen magnum. These vessels receive an additional blood supply at each cord segment from the lateral spinal arteries.

The central portion or gray matter of the cord is composed of the cell bodies of neurons and their dendrites. White matter (axons) surrounds the central gray and is divided into the anterior, lateral, and posterior columns or funiculi which are composed of ascending (sensory) and descending (motor) tracts (Figure 3-5).

The spinothalamic, spinocerebellar, and posterior columns are the primary ascending tracts. The lateral spinothalamic tracts convey sensations of pain and temperature from the spinal cord to the thalamus. The ventral spinothalamic tract carries light touch and pressure sensations to the thalamus. The posterior tracts conduct sensations of position, vibration, and deep touch or pressure to the thalamus and cerebrum. The dorsal and ventral spinocerebellar tracts carry proprioceptive impulses to the cerebellum.

The corticospinal, vestibulospinal, and reticulospinal are the primary descending tracts. Axons from the neurons (upper motor) in the cerebral cortex and brain stem cross over in the medulla to the opposite side and down the corticospinal (pyramidal) tracts to the anterior horn cells. Neurons located in the anterior horn cells are termed lower motor neurons. Their axons extend out from the nerves and synapses at the motor end plate with multiple peripheral muscle fibers to initiate upper and lower extremity movements. The vestibulospinal (extrapyramidal) tracts extend from the vestibular area of the brain stem to the cord and help maintain upright posture. The reticulospinal tracts also descend from the brain stem and connect with sympathetic ganglia to provide autonomic innervation.

Spinal Nerves

The 31 pairs of spinal nerves (eight cervical, 12 thoracic, five lumbar, five sacral, and one coccygeal) are part of the peripheral nervous system (PNS). While the upper cervical nerves have an almost horizontal course as they leave the intervertebral foramina, the course of the other spinal nerves becomes increasingly oblique, running almost vertical in the lumbar area and resembling a horse's tail (cauda equina).

Each nerve has a ventral and dorsal root (Figure 3-5). The ventral roots conduct efferent (motor) impulses to the skeletal muscles and through preganglionic sympathetic fibers of the autonomic nervous system. A myotome is a muscle group innervated by the motor fibers of the anterior root. The dorsal roots conduct afferent (sensory) impulses to the cord where they are transmitted to the brain via the ascending tracts. A dermatome is the area of skin innervated by the sensory fibers of the dorsal root of the spinal nerve (Figure 3-6).

By multiple subdivisions of these ventral and dorsal roots, nerves

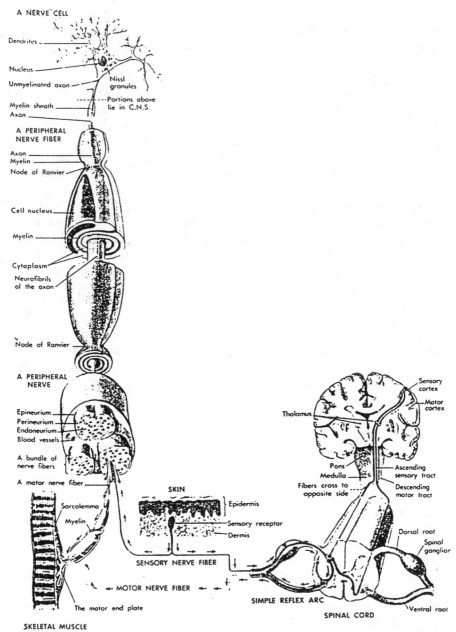

FIGURE 3-5 Structural highlights of the nervous system. (Guyton, A: *Structure and Function of the Nervous System* [2nd ed.] Philadelphia, W. B. Saunders, 1976.)

are distributed throughout the body. An intricate network of nerves is called a plexus. The cervical plexus consists of the first four cervical nerves and supplies the neck region. The phrenic nerve, which innervates the diaphragm, is an important branch of this plexus. The brachial plexus is formed from the fifth, sixth, seventh, and eighth cervical and first thoracic spinal nerves. It supplies the upper extremities. The radial, medial, and ulnar nerves are important branches of this plexus, providing innervation of the shoulder, arm,

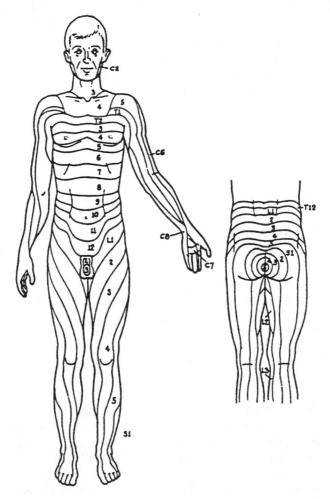

FIGURE 3-6 Dermatome chart. (Phillips, L., Ozer, M., Axelson, P., and Chizeck, H: *Spinal Cord Injury.* New York, Raven Press, 1987.)

forearm, wrist, and hand. The lumbar-sacral plexus is formed from the twelfth thoracic, the lumbar, and the sacral nerves; it supplies the pelvic and hip region and the lower extremities. The obturator, femoral, and sciatic nerves are its important branches. The thoracic nerves do not form a plexus, but pass out of the intercostal spaces between the ribs. They supply the thoracic and upper abdominal skin and musculature.

Reflex Arc

A reflex arc is comprised of a receptor (sense organ), an afferent neuron, an intercalated neuron, an efferent neuron, and an effector (skeletal muscle or gland). The impulse is initiated by stimulation of the receptor. The afferent neuron then transmits the impulse through the dorsal root of the spinal nerve to the spinal cord. There synapse occurs with the intercalated neuron, which then relays the impulse through the ventral root of the spinal nerve and the effector neuron to the effector (Figure 3-5).

AUTONOMIC NERVOUS SYSTEM (ANS)

The two divisions of the ANS, the sympathetic and the parasympathetic, act in an antagonistic manner to maintain a dynamic balance of the internal environment of the body. The fibers of the sympathetic (adrenergic) division originate in cell bodies in the lateral horns of the spinal cord between T1 and L2 (preganglionic neurons). They leave the cord through the anterior roots of the spinal nerves. After passing through small nerves called white rami, they synapse with neurons in the sympathetic chain (post-ganglionic neurons). Fibers from the post-ganglionic neurons may pass into the visceral sympathetic nerves that innervate the internal organs or they may return through the gray rami to the spinal nerves. Within these nerves they supply the blood vessels and sweat glands throughout the body. To provide sympathetic innervation above the thoracolumbar chain, fibers extend upward from the thoracic region into the neck and to the structures of the head. The lower abdomen and legs are supplied by fibers extending downward from the chain. Visceral sensory fibers pass with the sympathetic fibers through the sympathetic nerves where they travel into the spinal nerves. From there they enter the posterior horns of the cord gray matter and either cause the autonomic visceral reflexes or they transmit sensory impulses to the brain via the ascending tracts. Acetylcholine is the chemical transmitter at the preganglionic synapse and norepinephrine is at the postganglionic synapse.

Fibers from the parasympathetic (cholinergic) division originate mainly in the tenth cranial (vagus) nerve. A few also originate in the third, seventh, and ninth cranial nerves and in the sacral segments of the cord (S2-S4). The vagus nerve supplies parasympathetic fibers to the heart, lungs, and most of the organs of the abdomen. The other cranial nerves supply the head, and the sacral fibers supply the urinary bladder and distal parts of the colon. The cell bodies of the preganglionic fibers are in the brain stem or sacral cord. The fibers themselves pass all the way to the wall of the organ to be stimulated where they synapse with postganglionic neurons. Acetylcholine is the chemical transmitter at the pre and postganglionic synapses.

Table 3-3 outlines the main functions of each division of the ANS. The balanced harmony of these two divisions is disrupted during

**TABLE 3-3 Physiological Responses Resulting From
Autonomic Nervous System Stimulation**

Sympathetic, Adrenergic (thoracolumbar)		Parasympathetic, Cholinergic (craniosacral)
Increased	Mental Activity	—
Dilated	Pupils	Constricted
Decreased production	Salivary glands	Increased production
Increased production	Sweat glands	—
Dilated	Bronchioles	Constricted
Increased rate	Heart	Decreased rate
Dilated	Coronary arterioles	—
Increased	Blood glucose	—
Decreased	Stomach motility	Increases
Increased production	Adrenal glands	—
Decreased	Kidney output	Increased
Decreased production	Gastrointestinal glands	Increased production
Decreased	Intestinal motility	Increased
Constricted	Abdominal arterioles	Dilated
Decreased	Bladder tone	Increased
Increased tone	Anal, urethral sphincters	Relaxed
Ejaculation	Genitals	Erection
Constricted	Skin blood vessels	—
Vessels dilated	Skeletal muscles	Vessels dilated

times of physical and emotional stress when the sympathetic division assumes a dominant role. During periods of rest the parasympathetic division has a more dominant role, particularly in the digestive and elimination processes.

In addition to structural and physiological differences, the two autonomic divisions have differing pharmacologic effects. Sympathomimetic (adrenergic) drugs prepare the body for physiological stresses by acting on the organs in the same manner as the sympathetic nerves. Parasympathomimetic (cholinergic) drugs mimic the actions of the parasympathetic nervous system. Anticholinergic drugs, by negating the influence of the parasympathetic nervous system, have some of the same effects as adrenergic drugs. Adrenergic blockers, by negating the sympathetic nervous system response, have some of the same effects as the cholinergic drugs.

FUTURE IMPLICATIONS

A person who sustains damage to the nervous system experiences physiological/anatomical and behavioral/functional disruptions. Understanding of the specific mechanisms of neurological damage, dysfunction, and recovery is limited at present due to the complexity of the nervous system and the difficulty in separating the effects of intrinsic and extrinsic factors. A large number of research studies are being conducted in neurological physiology, pathophysiology, and rehabilitation. With increased knowledge gained from these studies it is hoped that existing management methods can be enhanced to more effectively reverse or inhibit neurological damage, to prevent disability-related complications, and to facilitate maximum physiological and psychological wellness for the person with a neurological disability. Subsequent chapters will discuss these topics in more detail as they relate to specific problems and disabilities.

REFERENCES

Duus, P. (1989). *Topical diagnosis in neurology: Anatomy, physiology, signs, symptoms* (2nd ed.). New York: Thieme Medical Publisher.

Fitzgerald, M. (1985). *Neuroanatomy basic and applied.* Oxford: Ballieri Tindall.

Guyton, A. (1976). *Structure and function of the nervous system* (2nd ed.). Philadelphia: W. B. Saunders Company.

Hickey, J. (1986). *The clinical practice of neurological and neurosurgical nursing* (2nd ed.). Philadelphia: J. B. Lippincott Company.

Marshall, S., Marshall, L., Vos, H., and Chestnut, R. (1990). *Neuroscience critical care: Pathophysiology and patient management.* Philadelphia: W. B. Saunders Company.

McClintic, J. (1985). *Physiology of the human body* (3rd ed.). New York: John Wiley and Sons.

Springer, S., and Deutsch, G. (1985). *Left brain right brain.* New York: W. H. Freeman.

Nursing Management of Problems Common to Neurorehabilitation

Neurogenic Bladder Management

4

OBJECTIVES

After completing this chapter, the reader will be able to:

- Describe the cognitive and physiological parameters for assessing the patient with the neurogenic bladder.
- Describe three categories of neurogenic bladder and the related pathophysiologies.
- Compare and contrast management interventions for these categories of dysfunction.
- Describe four potential complications related to neurogenic bladder and discuss appropriate preventive management.
- Discuss the psychological considerations related to neurogenic bladder management.

INTRODUCTION

The subject of neurogenic bladder management is multidimensional involving psychological, physiological, and educational parameters. Urological dysfunction can be an embarrassing, disrupting, and isolating problem for persons with neurological disabilities. In addition to the psychological ramifications, they are susceptible to life threatening physiological complications. Therefore, patient education is essential to help them regain a sense of control and confidence as well as to maximize bladder self-care abilities and prevent complications.

The goals of a nursing management plan include helping patients achieve and maintain balanced, functional bladders free from preventable complications, helping patients cope with the stress of urological dysfunction, and assisting them in learning to successfully manage their own regimes. The interventions required to achieve these goals are determined by each individual's neurological and urological status, pre-existing health problems, age, sex, psychosocial status, and discharge plan.

PHYSIOLOGY OF MICTURITION

Micturition is under both reflex and voluntary control. The micturition reflex is initiated when the quantity of urine in the bladder stimulates intramuscular sensory fibers. These fibers then send impulses via the pelvic (parasympathetic) nerve to the sacral reflex center located at the S2 to S4 level of the spinal cord. From there the impulses continue up the spinothalamic and posterior columns to the micturition centers in the frontal cortex and brain stem. Impulses from the brain stem move down the reticulospinal tract to the pelvic nerves. The pelvic nerves stimulate detrusor contraction, closure of

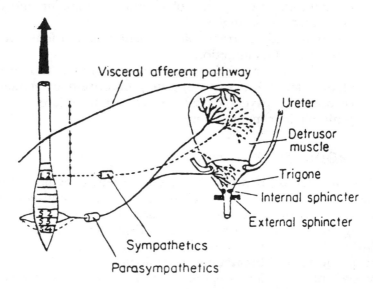

FIGURE 4-1 Urinary bladder and nervous pathways for the micturation reflex. (Guyton, A: *Function of the Human Body* [3rd ed.] Philadelphia: W. B. Saunders, 1969.)

the ureter orifices, and internal sphincter (bladder neck) relaxation. Voluntary control, maintained by contraction and relaxation of the external sphincter and pelvic floor muscles, is regulated by impulses moving from the frontal cortex down the corticospinal tract to the pudendal nerve. Sympathetic fibers are associated with bladder filling and urine storage. Adrenergic stimulation results in contraction at the bladder neck and outlet and detrusor relaxation (Figure 4-1).

PATHOPHYSIOLOGY

Bladder function can be impaired as a result of disruption of the neurological control mechanisms secondary to cortical or subcortical brain lesions, spinal cord lesions, peripheral nerve damage, or abnormalities in the autonomous innervation of the bladder wall (Tables 4-1 and 4-2). Age-related neurological changes can have the following effects on bladder function: Detrusor, bladder neck, and distal sphincter tone decreases; changes in brain cells or at ganglia or neurologic receptor sites in the lower urinary tract slow reaction time; and decreased kidney concentration ability increase volume of urine in the bladder. The following physical forces can also affect bladder function: Atrophic urethritis in the elderly; deterioration of urethral tone and intravesical changes secondary to long-term indwelling catheter use; urethral erosion, fistula and diverticula with repeated intermittent catheterization or long-term indwelling catheter.

Classification

Neurogenic bladders are categorize according to the type of dysfunction: Failure to store (associated with urge, stress, or reflex incontinence); failure to empty (associated with urinary retention and overflow incontinence); and combined dysfunction with a combination of retention and emptying problems (Table 4-3). Neurogenic bladders are also classified as uninhibited, reflex, mixed, autonomous, atonic, motor paralytic, and sensory paralytic (Table 4-1 and Figure 4-2). Alteration in urinary elimination patterns related to neurological dysfunction can occur in the form of urge, reflex, stress, functional, and overflow incontinence and urinary retention (Table 4-2).

TABLE 4-1 Neurogenic Bladder Classification and Related Pathophysiology

Classification	Description	Pathophysiology
Uninhibited	Normal bladder sensation, decreased capacity, urgency, frequency, incontinence, low post voiding residuals	Loss of cerebral inhibition of micturition reflex secondary to CVA, TBI, Alzheimer's disease, Parkinson's disease, or demyelinating plaques in brain
Reflex (spastic, hypertonic, automatic, upper motor neuron)	Impaired bladder sensation, decreased capacity, positive bulbocavernosus reflex, reflex incontinence	Spinal cord lesion above sacral reflex arc secondary to SCI, tumor, syringomyelia, or demyelinating plaques
Mixed	Elements of both upper and lower motor neuron bladder, i.e., weak or absent bladder sensation, hypotonic bladder with low pressure contractions, spastic external sphincter, variable residual volume and capacity, positive bulbocavernosus reflex	Spinal cord lesion above sacral reflex arc
Autonomous (hypotonic, lower motor neuron)	Absence of bladder sensation, flaccid bladder with increased capacity, negative bulbocavernosus reflex, overflow incontinence with high urine volumes	Damage to sacral reflex arc secondary to conus medullaris or cauda equina injury, demyelinating plaque, tumor or myelomeningocele
Atonic (areflexic)	Absence of bladder sensation and reflex, increased capacity, complete urinary retention	State of spinal shock following SCI
Motor paralytic	Normal bladder sensation, decreased tone, increased capacity, difficulty initiating urination	Lesions of ventral roots of S2 to S4 secondary to trauma, tumor, GBS, or polio
Sensory paralytic	Decreased bladder sensation leading to overdistention, high residuals, and incomplete emptying	Lesions of dorsal roots of S2 to S4 or peripheral neuropathy secondary to DM or pernicious anemia

**TABLE 4-2 Alteration in the Urinary Elimination Patterns
Related to Neurological Dysfunction**

Nursing Diagnosis	Pathophysiology
Urge incontinence	Detrusor instability related to neurological lesion above subcortical micturition center (uninhibited bladder) or in spinal cord above sacral reflex arc (reflex bladder); inflammatory conditions; bladder outlet obstruction
Reflex incontinence	Detrusor instability and detrusor sphincter dyssynergia related to spinal cord trauma, tumor, demyelinating plaque, or vascular disease
Stress incontinence	Intravesical pressure exceeding urethral closure pressure or decreased bladder outlet resistance related to DM neuropathy, spinal cord trauma or tumor, extensive abdominal and/or pelvic surgery
Functional incontinence	Alterations in cognition/behavior/functional ability related to Alzheimer's disease, TBI, biochemical changes
Total incontinence	Circumvention of normal sphincteric mechanism related to disease, trauma, surgery, or radiotherapy
Urinary retention	Deficient detrusor function, obstruction of bladder outlet, or both related to DM neuropathy, spinal shock, cauda equina injury, demyelinating plaques, polio, bladder neck hypertrophy, detrusor sphincter dyssynergia, urethral stricture, fecal impaction

Complications and Etiologies (Table 4-4)

Urinary Tract Infection (UTI)

This is the most frequently encountered complication in individuals with neurogenic bladders and can lead to renal damage if not carefully managed. Bladder distention with urine stasis is the most common cause of UTI. Distention and overstretching of the bladder tissue leads to a compromised blood supply to the cells. With the resulting ischemia there is a decrease in the number of leukocytes and antibacterial agents that are delivered to the area, therefore increasing the probability for infection. Other causative or contributing factors to infection development include poor instrumentation tech-

TABLE 4-3 Categories of Neurogenic Bladder Dysfunction

Category	Description	Symptoms
Failure to store	Hyperactive detrusor with uninhibited contraction	Reflex incontinence
Failure to empty	Weakened detrusor which is unable to exert enough force to expel all urine; spastic sphincter which interferes with complete emptying; simultaneous detrusor and sphincter contractions (detrusor sphincter dyssynergia)	Hesitancy, overflow incontinence, sensation, of incomplete emptying
Combined dysfunction	Active detrusor with tight sphincter	Urgency, nocturia, hesitancy, incontinence, sensation of incomplete emptying

nique, inadequate cleaning of equipment, decreased patient resistance, dehydration, and alkaline urine which potentiates bacteria growth. The severity of the infection is determined by the host's resistance, bladder and renal defense mechanisms, and the virulence of the infective organisms. In the male patient epididymitis may also develop from the same organisms causing the bladder infection.

Vesico-Ureteric Reflux

This condition occurs when increased intravesical pressure causes regurgitation of urine back up into the ureters. Chronic ascending infection and lower tract obstruction are the most common causes. A Grade I classification indicates minimal reflux into the lower ureter only. Grade II is complete reflux reaching the renal pelvis and calyces but without dilatation of the ureter, pelvis, or calyces. Grade III indicates marked reflux extending to the kidney with dilatation of the upper tract. Grade IV indicates massive reflux with pronounced hydronephrosis.

Hydronephrosis

This condition occurs as a result of an obstruction in a ureter or in the lower tract caused by calculi, a tumor, an enlarged prostate, a tight external sphincter, or an ascending infection which damages the ureter or the vesico-ureteric valve. There are five classifications

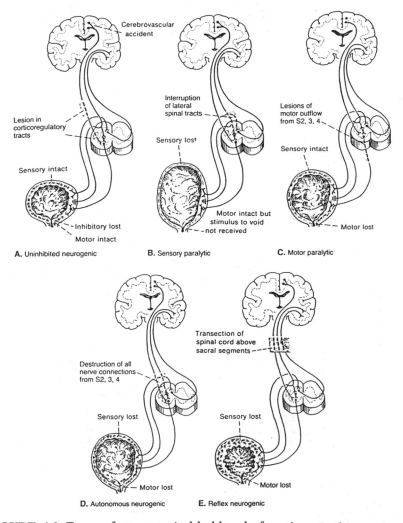

FIGURE 4-2 Types of neurogenic bladder dysfunction. (Luckmann, J., and Sorensen, K: *Medical–Surgical Nursing—A Psychophysiologic Approach* [3rd ed.] Philadelphia: W. B. Saunders, 1987.)

TABLE 4-4 Urinary Tract Complications

Pathology	Definition	Signs & Symptoms	Treatment	Prevention
Urinary tract infection	Infection of the bladder, kidneys, ureters, urethra. Causative or contributing factors: bladder distention and urine stasis, poor instrumentation technique, inadequate cleaning, decreased hose resistance, alkaline urine, low fluid intake	1. Rising temp 2. Hematuria 3. Foul smelling urine 4. Dysuria 5. Turbidity 6. Low back/flank pain 7. Elevated spasticity 8. Anorexia, fatigue 9. Diaphoresis	1. Increase fluid intake 2. Indwelling catheter 3. Antibiotics	1. Proper technique and consistent schedule with urine bladder catheterization 2. Regulate fluid intake and cath schedule to avoid bladder distention 3. Urinary antiseptic and Vit. C to lower pH
Calculi	Calcium or other mineral deposits lodged in any portion or urinary tract. Precipitating factors: infection, immobility, urine stasis	1. Hematuria 2. Turbidity 3. Low back/flank pain 4. Increased spasticity 5. Diaphoresis 6. Often accompanied infection	1. Cystolithopary 2. Percutaneous lithotripsy 3. ESWL 4. May pass stone sontaneously	1. Increase mobility 2. Lower urine stasis and residual 3. Increase fluid intake 4. Lower urine pH with Vit. C, cranberry juice

Hydronephrosis/ reflux	Dilation of the kidney and/or ureter. Causative factors: chronic ascending infection, lower tract obstruction	1. May be symptomatic 2. Often accompanied by infection	1. Indwelling catheter 2. Antibiotics 3. Avoid catheter irrigation and mechanical obstruction of catheter	1. Good bladder hygiene 2. Lower urine stasis and residuals 3. Lower sphincter resistance with medication, sphincterotomy
Detrusor sphincter dy-synergia	Hypotonic bladder and sphincter, simultaneous detrusor sphincter contraction Associated factor: incomplete SCI	1. Difficlty vaoiding 2. Increased residuals 3. Reflux	1. Lioresal 2. Dibenzyline 3. Minipress	—
Autonomic hyperreflexia	Exaggerated atonomic response to noxious stimulus below level of SCI Occurs in SCI about T6	1. Headache 2. Hypertension 3. Bradycardia 4. Diaphoresis 5. Congestion & chills 6. Blurred vision 7. Flushing above lesion	1. Raise head of bed 2. Remove noxious stimulus, i.e. empty distended bladder 3. Anticholinergic medication 4. Peripheral dilating medication	1. Regulation and monitoring of intake and output 2. Proper positioning of urine equipment 3. Measures to prevent infection and calculi
Penile scrotal fistula/urethral diverticula	Fistula at penoscrotal junction or urethral diverticula caused by indwelling catheter irritation	1. Difficulty inserting catheter 2. Often accompanied by infection	1. Remove indwelling catheter 2. May require suprapubic cystotomy	1. When indwelling cath required insert smallest size possible 2. Tape cath to lower abdomen in male, upper thigh in female

of hydronephrosis based on the severity of the problem. In Grade I the ureter is mildly dilated without obvious renal damage. Grade II indicates mild hydronephrosis. Grade III demonstrates a marked hydronephrosis. With Grade IV there is a large amount of dilatation of the kidney with obvious tissue strophy. In Grade V there is a large bag-like hydronephrosis with extensive tissue destruction.

Urinary Calculi

This condition results from an abnormal collection of mineral salts and other substances such as foreign bodies, cells, and bacteria. Ninety percent of urinary tract calculi are composed of calcium salts. One of the causes of calcium stone formation is from decalcification of bones as a result of non-weight-bearing. The calcium lost from the bones is filtered through the kidney filtration system. If the calcium-to-fluid ratio is high the calcium will come out of solution and crystallize. Urine stasis and infection from urea-splitting organisms can also be precipitating factors in stone formation. The size and location of the stones can vary from small, sandy particles in the bladder to large, staghorn calculi that occupy the entire renal pelvis.

Autonomic Hyperreflexia (Dysreflexia)

(See pages 136–137.) The stimulus that results in the exaggerated autonomic activity of this condition is most often a distended bladder. Urinary calculi, severe bladder infection, and bladder instrumentation are other stimuli that may initiate the response.

Peno-scrotal Fistula and Urethral Diverticula

These are complications that can result from using indwelling catheters that are too large, are left in too long, or are improperly positioned.

NURSING INTERVENTIONS

Assessment

Health History

- Site, type, completeness, and duration of the neurological condition.

- Type of motor, sensory, and autonomic dysfunction.
- Past and current urinary elimination difficulties.
- Past and current urinary tract complications.
- Episodes of autonomic hyperreflexia.
- Pre-morbid and current voiding and fluid intake pattern.
- Methods for initiating voiding.
- Diseases/conditions affecting or affected by GU status such as diabetes mellitus, cardiac disease, decubiti.
- Recurrent decubiti.
- Current medications.
- Psychosocial status.

Physical Assessment

- Observation of micturition.
- Flowsheet for voided and/or catheterized amounts and for frequency and amount of incontinent episodes.
- Observation of external genitalia for edema, sores, or discharge.
- Observation of surrounding skin for pustules or erosion.
- Palpation for prostate enlargement.
- Sitting balance and mobility.
- Ability to manipulate clothing and urinary equipment.
- Ability to recognize and verbalize desire to urinate.
- ability to learn management measures.

Note: During the history and physical assessment certain signs and symptoms of specific urological complications may be reported/ identified (Table 4-4).

Diagnostic Tests

- Blood tests to rule out electrolyte imbalances and renal impairment.
- Urodynamic studies: cystometrics to measure bladder and sphincter tone, filling pressure, and capacity; electromyography to diagnose detrusor sphincter dyssynergy; and urethral pressure profile to identify sites of urethral resistance and to measure pressure.
- Cystoscopy to determine presence of pathology through direct visualization.

- Cystourethrogram (voiding and retrograde) to observe the shape and capacity of the bladder and to rule out pathologies such as urethral diverticulum, reflux, tumors, and calculi.
- Intravenous pyelogram to observe upper urinary tract anatomy and to rule out renal and ureteric changes (IVP associated with high risk of renal failure in elderly).
- Isotope renography to demonstrate any upper tract disturbances such as reflux and hydronephrosis.
- Kidney/ureter/bladder radiograph to determine presence of calculi; to demonstrate bladder shape and presence of dilated ureters.
- Renal scintigraphy and arteriography to rule out urinary tract pathology and to demonstrate renal blood flow.
- Urine studies to determine presence of infection and renal impairment.

Nursing Diagnoses: Actual or Potential

1. Altered urinary elimination pattern: Incontinence, urgency, frequency, or retention related to neurological dysfunction.
2. Infection related to urinary stasis, distention, instrumentation techniques.
3. Urinary calculi related to immobility, infection, and decreased fluid intake.
4. Impaired skin integrity related to urinary incontinence.
5. Alterated comfort related to diagnostic and treatment procedures.
6. Self-care deficits: Urinary management related to sensory, motor, and/or cognitive deficits.
7. Disturbance in self-concept related to urological dysfunction and self-care deficits.
8. Anxiety related to threat to self-concept and urological dysfunction.
9. Ineffective individual coping related to inadequate information and urological dysfunction.
10. Social isolation related to embarrassment regarding urological condition, inaccessible bathrooms.

Expected Outcomes: Patient and/or Family

1. The individual achieves a routine of complete bladder elimination without incontinent episodes and renal function is preserved.

2. The individual is free of urinary tract complications.
3. The individual's skin integrity is maintained.
4. The individual copes with the discomfort of diagnostic and therapeutic procedures with minimum distress.
5. The individual engages in urinary self-care activities consistent with sensory, motor, and/or cognitive deficits.
6. The individual demonstrates the ability to perform or give instructions for urological techniques.
7. The individual experiences decreased anxiety and improved self-concept as evidenced by the individual's verbal report and/or body language.
8. The individual describes the factors that influence urinary elimination patterns and the management rationale.
9. The individual describes the potential problems related to neurogenic bladder dysfunction and strategies for preventing and coping with them.

Planning and Implementation

(Include the family, significant other, and/or caregiver in the teaching interventions.)

Failure to Store

For reflex incontinence establish an intermittent catheterization program (ICP) every 4 hours with progression dependent on catheterization volume and/or post void residuals. An ICP can maintain the health of the urinary system by preventing recurrent UTIs from urine stagnation and bladder distention, preventing kidney damage from bladder distention and ureteral reflux, relieving the patient of incontinence, and restoring bladder tone and function through periodic emptying. ICP is contraindicated when fluids cannot be restricted or in the presence of anatomical abnormalities such as meatal or urethral stenosis. Employ trigger techniques to facilitate reflex emptying in addition to ICP (or instead of ICP when post void residuals are less than 20 percent of bladder capacity). Assist the patient in learning self-catheterization and/or trigger techniques and fluid regulation.

For urge incontinence assist the patient in learning to maintain a timed voiding schedule starting every 2 hours and progressing to every 4 hours as feasible. Integrate behavior modification techniques when appropriate.

Identify factors associated with functional incontinence, such as altered environment or altered mentation, and design strategies to minimize these factors. Assess the medication regime to prevent idiopathic incontinence.

Select appropriate urinary containment devices for incontinence such as condom devices and incontinence briefs. There are female external devices available but adherence and skin irritation remain major problems. Assist the patient in learning correct application, removal, and skin care techniques.

Promote storing by administering prescribed medication to increase urethral and bladder neck resistance (ephedrine/Ephedsol, phenylephrine/Sudafed); to decrease bladder contractility and spasticity (oxybutynin chloride/Ditropan, flavoxate/Urispas, imipramine/Tofranil, hyoscyamine/Cystospaz, propantheline bromide/Pro Banthine). Observe and record patient response. Take precautions to minimize side effects of the medications. Assist the patient in learning the medication purpose, dosage, schedule, side effects, and precautions.

Failure to Empty

For urinary retention establish an ICP every 4 hours with progression dependent on catheterization volume and patient's fluid intake. Assist the patient in learning fluid regulation, self-catheterization techniques, and/or techniques to facilitate voiding (with the urologist approval) such as the Valsalva or crede maneuver or the anal sphincter stretch.

Insert an indwelling catheter only when other strategies are inappropriate as with ureteral reflux. To prevent a penoscrotal fistula or urethral diverticula, select smallest size catheter with the smallest balloon whenever possible and tape the catheter to the patient's abdomen (male) or upper thigh (female). (Note: An indwelling catheter may also be required when fluid restriction is contraindicated for the patient with incontinence.) Assist the patient in learning catheter insertion and management techniques and the importance of increased fluid intake (3000-4000 cc qd).

Promote emptying by administering prescribed medication to enhance bladder contractility (bethanecol hydrochloride/Urecholine); to increase relaxation of urethral smooth muscle and decrease outflow resistance (phenoxybenzamine/Dibenzyline or prazosin/Minipress); to increase relaxation of striated external sphincter (diazepam/Valium, baclofen/Lioresal, dantrolene sodium/Dantrium). Observe and record patient response. Take precautions to minimize the side effects of the medication. Assist the patient in learning the medication purpose, dosage, schedule, side effects, and precautions.

Complications

Refer to Table 4-4.

Assist the patient in learning measures to prevent and treat urinary tract complications.

Surgical Interventions

The urethral prosthesis is designed to simulate normal action of the perineum and sphincter by closing off the urethra. Two rod-shaped tubes are inserted parallel to the urethra. These rods are connected to a pressure device in the groin that allows the individual to inflate (close) and deflate (open) the prosthesis. This eliminates the daily need for catheterization. For this to be a satisfactory alternative, the individual needs to have enough upper extremity strength and dexterity to perform transfers, undress, and manipulate the prosthesis. Assist the patient in learning proper management techniques.

With the continent vesicotomy an anterior flap of the bladder wall is formed into a valve-like intussusception which leads to a stoma on the anterior abdominal wall. It is a reversible procedure. The potential complications include suture dehiscence, stomal stenosis, infection, and calculi. Assist the patient in learning management techniques and how to identify complications.

The objective of a transurethral resection and external sphincterotomy (TURES) is to diminish bladder neck and sphincter resistance to urine outflow. The criteria for surgery are based on a variety of clinical and diagnostic parameters including the presence of severe detrusor sphincter dyssynergia, vesico-ureteric reflux, high residuals with hyperreflexia, or upper tract changes with sustained high intravesical pressure and spastic sphincter. Because permanent incontinence is one result, the sphincterotomy should not be performed on anyone who has the potential for more neurological return. Assist the patient in understanding the procedure and follow-up care that is required.

Extracorporeal shock-wave lithotripsy (ESWL) uses shock waves generated outside the body to break up kidney stones inside the body without harming the kidneys or nearby organs. The advantages over traditional kidney surgery include a shorter hospital stay, reduced incidence of pain, and a decreased risk of complications. Percutaneous lithotripsy is another procedure that may be used if the patient is not a candidate for ESWL. In this procedure the kidney stones are removed through a catheter that has been introduced into the kidney collecting system through an incision over the site. Assist the patient in understanding the procedures and the related management measures.

Psychological Considerations

Maintain the patient's privacy and dignity during all procedures.

Provide time and a supportive environment in which the patient can express fears and frustrations regarding urological problems. Assist him/her in enhancing coping skills.

Be sensitive to the patient's cultural background and value systems and how these may impact on the treatment plan.

Collaborate with the patient to develop a home bladder management program appropriate to his/her lifestyle and abilities.

FUTURE IMPLICATIONS

Research has been directed at efforts to maximize the effectiveness and decrease the complications related to the traditional approaches for neurogenic bladder management and to develop improved management techniques that will further decrease the probability of complications and increase the patient's physical and psychological freedom from urological concerns. The following provide examples demonstrating both the progress and the continuing problems with these efforts.

1. Biofeedback has been used with moderate success to increase sensory awareness of bladder filling.
2. Electrical stimulation has been used with moderate success to increase bladder tone and to facilitate timed and complete bladder emptying.
3. The artificial sphincter has been used with variable success to control incontinence and retention. A high incidence of infec-

tion remains an ongoing concern with this management method.

4. Women trying the newer female urinary collecting devices continue to experience problems with adherence and skin irritation.

5. Studies have continued to support the contention that clean technique with a consistent ICP can be as effective as sterile technique for reducing the incidence of UTI, as bacteria introduced into the bladder are flushed out by periodic complete emptying and patients are more likely to maintain a consistent catheterization schedule with the less complicated approach.

6. ESWL has reduced the pain and risk of complications and shortened hospital stays for individuals with urinary calculi.

Decreased urologically-related mortality and morbidity rates in the neurologically impaired population is the most striking and encouraging evidence of the ongoing progress being made in the areas of diagnosis, prevention, and treatment.

REFERENCES

Abrams, P. (1985). Detrusor instability and bladder outlet obstruction. *Neurourology and Urodynamics, 4*:317–328.

Abrams, P., Feneley, R., and Tarrens, M. (1988). *Urodynamics.* Berlin: Springer-Verlag.

Ader, K., Pierce, L., and Salter, J. (1990). Urinary tract infections: Quality assurance rehabilitation nursing perspectives. *Rehabilitation Nursing, 15*(4):193–196.

Bradley, W. (1986). Physiology of micturition. In P. Walsh, R., Gitles, A. Perlmutter, and T. Stamey. *Campbell's urology.* Philadelphia: W. B. Saunders Company.

Cardenas, D., Kelly, E., and Mayo, M. (1985). Manual stimulation of reflex voiding after SCI. *Archives of Physical Medicine and Rehabilitation, 66*(7):459–462.

Chaussy, C. (Ed.). (1986). *Extracorporeal shock-wave lithotripsy: Technical concepts, experimental research, and clinical application.* New York: Eastern Paralyzed Veteran's Association.

Cioschi, H. (1987). Alterations in urinary elimination. In Rehabilitation Nursing Foundation. *Application of Rehabilitation Concepts to Nursing Practice* (2nd Ed.). Evanston, IL: Rehabilitation Nursing Foundation.

Gray, M. and Broadwell, D. (1986). Genitourinary disease. In J. Thompson, G. McFarland, J. Hirsch, S. Tucker, and A. Bowers. *Clinical nursing.* St. Louis: C.V. Mosby Company.

Hanak, M. (1986). *Patient and family education.* New York: Springer Publishing Company.

McGurie, E., and Savastano, J. (1985). Stress incontinence and detrusor instability/urge incontinence. *Neurourology and Urodynamics, 4*:313–316.

Mumma, C. (Ed.). (1987). *Rehabilitation nursing: Concepts and practice.* Evanston: Rehabilitation Nursing Foundation.

Oliver, L. (1990). Neurogenic bladder. In K. Jeter, N. Faller, and C. Norton (Eds.). *Nursing for Continence.* Philadelphia: W. B. Saunders Co.

Pires, M. (1990). Promoting continence for the physically impaired. In K. Jeter, N. Faller, and C. Norton (Eds.). *Nursing for Continence.* Philadelphia: W. B. Saunders Co.

Ruge, C. (1986). Shockwave treatment for kidney stones. *American Journal of Nursing,* (1987), *86*(4):400.

Voith, A. (1988). Alterations in urinary elimination: Concepts, research, and practice. *Rehabilitation Nursing, 13*(3):122–131.

Neurogenic Bowel Management

5

OBJECTIVES

After completing this chapter, the reader will be able to:

- Describe the cognitive and physiological parameters for assessing the patient with neurogenic bowel.
- Discuss five classifications of neurogenic bowel and the related pathophysiologies.
- Discuss the management modalities and special considerations for each type of neurogenic bowel.
- Identify three potential complications related to neurogenic bowel and describe the appropriate preventive management.
- Discuss the psychological considerations related to neurogenic bowel management.

INTRODUCTION

Bowel incontinence resulting from neurogenic dysfunction is a frequently encountered consequence of a neurological disability. This and related bowel problems can have a devastating emotional impact on the individuals experiencing them. Elimination is usually a very private concern and an embarrassing subject to discuss. In addition to the psychological ramifications, bowel dysfunction can result in some uncomfortable and potentially serious medical complications. Therefore, patient education is essential to help each individual regain a sense of control and confidence as well as to maximize bowel self-care abilities and prevent complications.

The goals of a nursing management program include assisting the patients in achieving and maintaining a schedule of predictable, complete evacuations without the complications of incontinence, constipation, impaction, and diarrhea; helping patients cope with the stress of bowel dysfunction; and assisting them in learning how to successfully manage their own routines.

PHYSIOLOGY OF DEFECATION

Defecation results form the action of the defecation reflex augmented by the sacral cord reflex. These reflexes can be inhibited or facilitated by voluntary control. With the defecation reflex, feces in the rectum distend the rectal wall. This initiates afferent impulses that spread through the myenteric plexus, initiating peristaltic waves in the descending colon and sigmoid, and forcing feces toward the anus. As the peristaltic wave approaches the anus, the internal anal sphincter relaxes. When the external sphincter is voluntarily relaxed, defecation occurs.

Because the defecation reflex is extremely weak, it is fortified by another reflex involving the sacral cord segments and the autonomic nervous system. Rectal distention stimulates the afferent fibers which transmit impulses to and from the sacral reflex center via the pelvic (parasympathetic) nerve. These impulses, traveling back to the rectum, greatly intensify the peristaltic waves, increase abdominal pressure, relax the internal sphincter, and make the defecation reflex more effective (Figure 5-1).

With the voluntary pathway, awareness of defecation occurs when increased peristalsis and internal sphincter relaxation stimulate the pudendal nerve, which sends impulses up the spinothalamic tract of the spinal cord to the brain. The brain then sends impulses back down the corticospinal tracts to initiate the valsalva maneuver, which increases intra-abdominal pressure, increases straightening and elongation of the colon, moves the feces into the rectum, and relaxes the internal and external sphincters. An alternative action from the voluntary pathway is inhibition of the defecation reflexes through inhibition of the external sphincter. Sympathetic stimulation (T6-L3) can also inhibit defecation by decreasing peristalsis and contracting the internal anal sphincter.

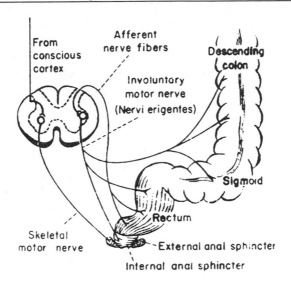

FIGURE 5-1 Anatomy of the defecation reflex. (Guyton, A: *Function of the Human Body* [3rd ed.] Philadelphia: W. B. Saunders, 1969.)

Many factors can affect the elimination pattern of an individual. These include impaired cognition, which affects voluntary control and the ability to learn the bowel routine; impaired balance and stability, which affects functional ability; impaired motor control, which affects functional ability and can affect defecation directly if the diaphragm, abdominal, and pelvic muscles are involved; and food and fluid imbalances (low fiber and fluid). Medications can affect elimination directly or indirectly. Magnesium-based antacids can cause diarrhea; aluminum-based antacids can cause constipation; anticholinergics and narcotics can cause constipation secondary to decreased GI motility; and diuretics can cause constipation secondary to dehydration. A high level of stress can also cause constipation by decreasing GI motility secondary to sympathetic stimulation.

PATHOPHYSIOLOGY

Bowel function can be adversely affected by preexisting diseases such as diverticulitis, colitis, and Crohn's Disease. Bowel function can also be impaired as a result of disruption in the neurological control mechanisms secondary to cortical or subcortical brain lesions, spinal cord lesions, an peripheral nerve damage.

Classification

There are five classifications of neurogenic bowel. Each is characterized by the functional ability and the related characteristics of that particular bowel type (see Table 5-1).

TABLE 5-1 Neurogenic Bowel Classification and Related Pathophysiology

Classification	Description	Pathophysiology
Uninhibited (upper motor neuron)	Normal perianal sensation, impaired awareness of urge, sphincter intact, intact bulbocavernosus reflex, urgency, potential for incontinence	Disruption of facilitory and inhibitory signals due to brain damage at cortical or subcortical level 2° to CVA, TBI, Alzheimer's disease, tumor, or MS
Reflex (spastic, hypertonic, automatic, upper motor neuron)	Impaired perianal sensation, impaired awareness of urge, intact bulbocavernosus reflex and sphincters, reflex incontinence	Neurological damage above sacral reflex center 2° to SCI or MS
Areflexic (autonomous, lower motor neuron)	Diminished or absent perianal sensation, awareness of urge, internal sphincter intact, absent external sphincter response, absent bulbocavernosus reflex, incontinence 2° to flaccid external sphincter	Neurological damage to sacral reflex arc 2° to conus medullaris, cauda equina, or peripheral nerve injury, myelomeningocele, MS, or tumor below S2-S4
Sensory paralytic	Diminished or absent perianal sensation, impaired awareness of urge, diminished bulbocavernosus reflex, constipation 2° to decreased awareness of urge, incontinence rare except in advanced stages of precipitating disease	Damage to dorsal roots of S2-S4 2° to DM, tabes dorsalis
Motor paralytic	Normal perianal sensation, awareness of urge, sphincters intact, bulbocavernosus reflex absent, constipation 2° to decreased bowel tone	Damage to ventral roots of S2-S4 2° to polio, trauma, or tumor

NURSING INTERVENTIONS

Assessment

Health History

- Site, type, completeness, and the duration of the neurological condition.
- Type of motor, sensory, and autonomic dysfunction.
- Type of reflex activity present.
- Pre-existing GI pathology/previous surgery.
- Previous and current elimination patterns.
- Current evacuation facilitation methods and effectiveness.
- Nutritional and fluid intake pattern.
- Factors adversely affecting nutritional status such as dysphagia or dental problems.
- Current medication.
- Psychosocial status.

Physical Assessment

- Presence or absence of bowel sounds.
- Presence or absence of perianal sensation.
- Presence or absence of bulbocavernosus reflex.
- Flowsheet recording the results of bowel stimulation and incontinent episodes and relation of diet and activity to incontinent episodes.
- Observation of perianal area and surrounding skin for signs of irritation or breakdown and presence of internal or external hemorrhoids.
- Sitting balance and mobility.
- Ability to manipulate clothing and equipment.
- Ability to interpret and communicate need to defecate.
- Ability to learn bowel management program.

During the physical assessment certain signs and symptoms of specific bowel complications may be identified (Table 5-2).

Diagnostic Tests

An abdominal radiograph may be taken if there is a suspicion of a probable impaction. Otherwise, formal GI testing is usually not per-

TABLE 5-2 Neurogenic Bowel Complications

Complication	Symptoms	Etiology
Constipation and impaction	Loss of appetite, nausea, diaphoresis, headache, abdominal discomfort/ distention, decreased bowel sounds, infrequent, irregular evacuation pattern	Decreased mobility, muscle weakness, inadequate diet, decreased bowel tone, medications
Diarrhea	Loss of appetite, nausea, diaphoresis, abdominal cramping if sensation present, hyperactive bowel sounds, frequent watery stools	Dietary changes, antibiotics, virus
Autonomic hyper-reflexia	Subjective: headache, diaphoresis, chills, nasal congestion, chest pressure, nervousness Objective: hypertension, bradycardia, diaphoresis, flushed face	Bowel impaction, instrumentation, disimpaction
Paralytic ileus	Abdominal distention, absent bowel sounds	Occurs within 24-48 hours after SCI and other neurological trauma possible 2° to sudden cessation of autonomic innervation

formed unless there is evidence of other GI pathology unrelated to the neurogenic dysfunction.

Nursing Diagnoses: Actual or Potential

1. Alteration in bowel elimination: Constipation related to immobility, diet, medications, or impaired reflex center; incontinence related to impaired voluntary control; diarrhea related to diet or medications.
2. Altered comfort related to constipation, impaction, or diarrhea.
3. Impaired skin integrity related to incontinence.

4. Self-care deficit: Bowel management related to sensory, motor, and/or cognitive deficits.
5. Disturbance in self-concept related to bowel dysfunction and self-care deficits.
6. Anxiety related to threat to self-concept and bowel dysfunction.
7. Ineffective individual coping related to self-care deficits and loss of bowel control.
8. Social isolation related to embarrassment regarding bowel dysfunction, inaccessible bathrooms.

Expected Outcomes: Patient and/or Family

1. The individual's elimination pattern is stabilized.
2. The individual remains comfortable and free of bowel incontinence, constipation, and diarrhea.
3. The individual's skin integrity is maintained.
4. The individual engages in bowel management self-care activities consistent with sensory, motor, and/or cognitive deficits.
5. The individual demonstrates ability to perform or give instructions for bowel management techniques.
6. The individual experiences decreased anxiety and depression, and improved self-concept as evidenced by the individual's verbal report and/or body language.
7. The individual describes the factors that influence bowel elimination patterns and the management rationale.
8. The individual describes the potential problems related to bowel dysfunction and strategies for preventing and coping with them.

Planning and Implementation

(Include the family, significant other, and/or caregiver in the teaching interventions.)

Using the information obtained from the health history and physical assessment, a program can be designed for each individual based on present elimination patterns, eating habits and preferences, activity level, lifestyle, support system, coping abilities, and the type of disability and how this has affected functional abilities, plus the goals that have been mutually defined and the potential level of patient cooperation. This information is then integrated into the following basic components of a neurogenic bowel management program.

Diet

Implement the necessary diet and fluid intake modifications to insure that the individual is receiving an adequate amount of bulk, roughage, and fluid. Bulk is needed for the production of well-formed stools. Foods high in bulk include whole grain products such as bran, whole wheat, and cornmeal. Ingestion of large quantities of bulk foods without adequate fluid intake (approximately 2000 cc per day) for lubrication can create impaction problems. Stimulants will help intensify the peristaltic action of the bowel. Roughage in the form of fresh fruits and vegetables provides some of this stimulation as well as bulk. Particularly helpful for their stimulating effects are prunes, figs, and dates. Spicy foods, caffeine, and alcohol also provide an irritant type of stimulation. Foods that tend to constipate include such items as white rice, white potatoes, white pasta, cheese, and chocolate.

Timing

Establish a regular schedule of rectal stimulation and/or toileting. (Rectal stimulation increases colon peristalsis and produces a more complete emptying of the lower bowel. It may be contraindicated in patients with cardiac conditions.) When possible, take advantage of the gastrocolic reflex which occurs 15 to 30 minutes after each meal. Use the same time frame as the individual's previous evacuation pattern if possible. In establishing an effective schedule, consideration must be given to the individual's lifestyle and the amount of assistance that may be needed.

Positioning

Facilitate evacuation by having the individual in a position that is anatomically conducive for elimination, either sitting with the knees higher than the hips or left sidelying. Augment weakened or paralyzed abdominal muscles by use of abdominal massage, an abdominal binder, and supporting the individual in a leaning over position. If some abdominal muscle strength is present and there are no cardiovascular contraindications, encourage the individual to use the abdominal muscles to bear down.

Activity

Encourage increased activity appropriate to the individual's tolerance and functional level to counteract the constipating effects of immobility. Work with the physical therapist and occupational therapist to facilitate maximum mobility and independence in bowel management activities.

Medications

If bowel results are inadequate and inconsistent in spite of implementing corrective dietary, scheduling, activity, and positioning measures, medications such as stool softeners, gentle stimulants, and bulk laxatives may be needed. (Note: Adequate fluid intake is required when using stool softeners and bulk laxatives.) Harsh laxatives and enemas should not be used on a regular basis as they can lead to long-term management problems.

Other medications can also have an effect on the function of a neurogenic bowel. For example, narcotics and antacids containing aluminum hydroxide can be constipating. Anticholinergic and sympathomimetic medications can also decrease GI motility. Antibiotics can decrease the normal GI flora which can result in diarrhea. It may be necessary to re-evaluate the medication regime if any of these medications are creating problems and determine if adjustments can be made to reduce or eliminate the bowel disrupting effects.

Managing and Preventing Complications

Paralytic ileus: Insert a nasogastric tube (NGT), connect it to low suction, and keep the patient NPO until bowel sounds return.

Constipation: Review fluid intake (increase as needed) and diet (increase fiber, decrease constipating foods). Assess need for medication changes (decrease anticholinergics, increase softeners and/or stimulants). Review schedule, activity, positioning, and stimulation techniques and make changes as needed.

Impaction/obstruction: Check bowel sounds. Palpate abdomen. Assist in obtaining an abdominal flat plate. Administer oral laxatives and enemas. With complete obstruction the patient may require temporary NGT insertion and gastric decompression to prevent vomiting and subsequent aspiration until the obstruction is eliminated.

Diarrhea: Review with the patient any dietary factors that may have caused or contributed to the problem. Encourage adjustments as needed and review the rationale with the patient. If diarrhea is related to antibiotic therapy, diet adjustments and the addition of unsweetened yogurt may be helpful. Provide scrupulous skin care after each bowel movement. If the diarrhea is severe, additional causes may need to be explored. Fluid and electrolyte replacements may also be needed.

Autonomic hyperreflexia (see pages 136–137): Assist the patient to a partial sitting position. Insert a local anesthetic cream into the rectum 10 minutes prior to disimpacting. Monitor vital signs frequently as the stimulation of the disimpaction process may further exacerbate the symptoms and raise the blood pressure. Oral laxatives may be needed to move a high impaction. Anticholinergic or vasodilating drugs may be necessary to reduce symptoms and ease the patient's discomfort. Assist the patient in learning the symptoms and causes of hyperreflexia and prevention measures such as maintaining a well regulated bowel routine.

The preceding guidelines are applicable to each type of neurogenic bowel. However, the management emphasis will vary slightly. For example, the person with a reflex bowel will be more responsive to the stimulation of a suppository or digital than will the person with an autonomous, sensory, or motor paralytic bowel. Those individuals are likely to have more difficulty establishing a successful routine and need to put additional emphasis on diet and intra-abdominal maneuvers while maintaining a regular evacuation schedule. Scheduling remains a crucial factor for the person with an uninhibited bowel, but rather than focusing on stimulation of the reflex arc as with the reflex bowel, the focus is on stimulating conscious awareness and control of the reflex activity. A behavior modification approach may be beneficial in this situation.

Psychological Considerations

Maintain the patient's privacy and dignity during the bowel routine.

Provide private time within and a supportive environment in which the patient can express and explore fears and frustrations regarding elimination problems. Assist him/her in enhancing coping skills.

Be sensitive to the patient's cultural background and value systems and how these may impact on the treatment plan.

Assist the patient in regaining a sense of control by learning his or her body's responses to the variables that contribute to a successful bowel program (diet, timing, positioning, activity, medications) and how to manage these variables to prevent and deal with complications.

FUTURE IMPLICATIONS

In spite of adhering to diet, scheduling, positioning, and medication guidelines, embarrassing episodes of incontinence or uncomfortable and potentially dangerous episodes of constipation and impaction occur too frequently for many people with neurogenic bowel. One promising area of research is with biofeedback and electrical stimulation. The goal of this research is to facilitate fecal retention and evacuation through neuromuscular re-education. At this point studies have been limited to individuals with CVA. Further research will be needed with CVA patients and with other disability groups before this method can be considered an acceptable bowel management method. At this time education and support remain the most important nursing measures for helping the person with a neurological disability achieve and maintain a successful bowel program.

REFERENCES

Buchanan, L. and Narvoczenski, D. (Eds.). (1987). *Spinal cord injury: Concepts and management approaches.* Baltimore: Williams and Wilkins.

Cisschi, H. (1987). Alterations in bowel elimination. In Rehabilitation Nursing Foundation. *Application of Rehabilitation Concepts in Nursing Practice* (2nd ed.). Evanston: Rehabilitation Nursing Foundation.

Hanak, M. (1986). *Patient and family education: Teaching programs for managing chronic disease and disability.* New York: Springer Publishing Company.

Hickey, J. (1986). *The clinical practice of neurological and neurosurgical nursing* (2nd ed.). Philadelphia: J.P. Lippincott Company.

Mumma, C. (Ed.). (1987). *Rehabilitation nursing: Concepts and practice* (2nd ed.). Evanston: Rehabilitation Nursing Foundation.

Sanders, K. (1989). Colonic movements: A rhythmic duet of two pacemakers. *Paraplegia News*, Special Section: 3–4.

Staas, W., and La Mantia, J. (1984). Bowel function and control. In Ruskin, A. (Ed.). *Current therapy in physiatry*. Philadelphia: W. B. Saunders Company.

Stone, J. (1989). Gastrointestinal problems after SCI: Challenge for the 1990's. *Paraplegia News*, Special Section: 2–3.

Dysphagia Management   6

OBJECTIVES

After completing this chapter, the reader will be able to:

- Describe the cognitive and physiological parameters for assessing the patient with dysphagia.
- Discuss the neurological disorders and cranial nerve impairments associated with dysphagia.
- Outline the steps for managing the patient with dysphagia and discuss the rationale for each step.
- Discuss psychological considerations related to dysphagia management.

INTRODUCTION

The term dysphagia refers to a dysfunction or difficulty in swallowing. If not managed effectively, dysphagia can lead to the serious and potentially life-threatening complications of aspiration pneumonia, fluid and electrolyte imbalances, and severe nutritional depletion. Successful management can be difficult and challenging. Some individuals with this condition may not be able to understand the instructions involved in training or the reasons for following specific guidelines. Others, out of frustration and impatience, may put themselves in danger by ingesting foods and fluids that they cannot safely and effectively swallow.

A successful management plan addresses these cognitive and psychological factors as well as the physiological factors. A coordinated team effort between speech pathology, occupational therapy, nutritional therapy, and nursing is essential in assisting the patient to achieve the goals of the dysphagia management program: (a) preventing aspiration, (b) regaining the ability to swallow safely and effectively, and (c) maintaining an optimum nutritional status. Family members need to be involved in all aspects of the treatment and educational plan so they do not inadvertently jeopardize the patient's health by offering foods and fluids that he or she is not capable of swallowing.

PHYSIOLOGY OF SWALLOWING (DEGLUTITION)

The primary physiological goals in the swallowing process are (a) formation of a bolus, (b) intact bolus propulsion, (c) prevention of food and fluid from being aspirated, (d) rapid movement of the bolus through the pharynx to minimize the suspension of respiration time, (e) prevention of gastric reflux during esophageal emptying, and (f) the clearance of bolus residue from the pharyngeal esophageal tract. A normal swallow requires an awareness of the process, functional facial, intraoral, and laryngeal muscles, and an intact nervous system. The swallowing sequence occurs in three stages—the oral, pharyngeal, and esophageal phases—and takes about 5 to 9 seconds.

The oral stage is initiated when food is ingested, chewed, lubricated, and moved to the rear of the mouth by the tongue. After this largely voluntary step, a reflexive swallow propels the food bolus into the pharynx. This reflex occurs in response to stimulation of the taste and touch receptors in the oropharynx. Chewing can also stimulate the reflex. The motor component of this stage if mediated through cranial nerve CNV (trigeminal nerve), CNVII (facial nerve), and CNXII (hypoglossal nerve). Afferent function is mediated through CNV, CNIX (glossopharyngeal nerve), and CNX (vagus nerve).

The pharyngeal stage begins when the bolus enters the pharynx and ends as the bolus is propelled into the esophagus. This phase of swallowing is involuntary and totally reflexive. It is initiated by touch receptors in the pharynx which stimulate CNIX. This nerve transmits impulses to the medullary center which, in turn, outputs motor impulses via CNX, which mediates various protective and propulsive movements. Food is prevented from entering the respira-

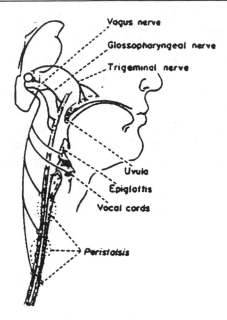

FIGURE 6-1 Anatomy of the Swallowing Mechanism. (Guyton, A: *Function of the Human Body* [3rd ed.] Philadelphia: W. B. Saunders, 1969.)

tory system through velopharyngeal closure, larynx elevation, and glottis closure. Additional motions result in an increase in pharyngeal pressure, which augments the pharyngeal contractions to move the bolus to the esophagus.

The final stage, the esophageal stage, begins immediately after the larynx is lowered, the glottis reopened, and the upper esophageal sphincter contracted to seal off the upper end of the esophagus. The food bolus is then propelled to the lower digestive tract by peristaltic movements and the relaxation of the lower esophageal sphincter. Efferent innervation originates from CNX. This phase of swallowing is also involuntary and reflexive.

Some of the primary anatomical features of the swallowing mechanism are illustrated in Figure 6-1.

PATHOPHYSIOLOGY

Dysphagia occurs most frequently in those individuals who have experienced disease or trauma to the central nervous system. (The mechanical disorders affecting swallowing are not addressed in this chapter.) The presentation of the disorder can vary considerably depending on which stages are affected. Impairments in the innervation of facial and tongue muscles will disturb the oral stage of swallowing. Persons with oral stage disorders tend to drool and pocket food in their mouths. Those with pharyngeal stage disorders usually exhibit a hypernasal voice quality and nasal regurgitation of fluids resulting from inadequate velopharyngeal closure. They may experience aspiration due to an absence of the gag reflex, a failure of the esophageal sphincter to relax, or a failure of the vocal cords to close. Individuals with esophageal stage innervation disorders frequently experience regurgitation, pain, and aspiration as a result of upper and/or lower esophageal sphincter dysfunction.

The following acquired neurological disorders frequently cause dysphagia:

Stroke syndromes, particularly brain stem strokes, may cause vocal cord and palate paralysis, laryngeal weakness due to CNIX, CNX, and medulla involvement. Strokes may also affect swallowing by damaging CNV, VII, and XII (oral stage) and by interrupting the corticospinal pathways and reflex connections.

Traumatic brain injury (TBI) can cause swallowing problems similar to those seen in various stroke syndromes if there has been damage to any of the cranial nerves involved with swallowing or any of the brain stem structures involved with processing and coordinating impulse transmission.

Parkinson's disease may result in a delay in the initiation of swallowing, irregular movement of the epiglottis, decreased esophageal peristalsis and autonomic dysfunction such as sialorrhea.

Amyotrophic lateral sclerosis (ALS) may cause CNIX and CNX dysfunction with subsequent pharyngeal and laryngeal impairment as well as CNXII dysfunction with tongue weakness. There may also be upper esophageal sphincter impairment.

Advanced multiple sclerosis (MS) may affect various stages of the swallowing process depending on the location of the neuropathology.

NURSING INTERVENTIONS

Assessment

Health History

- Type of neurological damage
- Episodes of nasopharyngeal regurgitation.
- Episodes of aspiration.
- Diagnosis of aspiration pneumonia.
- Episodes of heartburn after eating.
- Recent weight loss.
- Current medications (Some sedatives, antispasmodics, anticholinergics, and tranquilizers can affect swallowing.)

Physical Assessment

(It is recommended that the physical assessment be performed in collaboration with the speech pathologist whenever possible. Psychometric screening may also be needed to assess perceptual and language function.)

- Mental status and ability to cooperate and follow instructions.
- Presence of motor planning disorders.
- Ability to perform motor tasks and maintain control of the head.
- Facial and mastication muscles strength and function.
- Condition of natural teeth or dentures and effect on chewing.
- Presence of pathological reflexes of sucking, biting, moving the head and lips in the directions of the stimulus, and spontaneous mouth opening.
- Presence of sialorrhea
- Status of the oral mucosa: Presence of lesions, excessive dryness, or tenacious mucus.
- Position and appearance of the uvula and the palatal arch.
- Presence of gag reflex and the effectiveness of the velopharyngeal closure.
- Tongue appearance and strength.
- Presence of laryngeal movement during a test swallow. (A test

swallow should not be performed if the patient does not have an adequate cough reflex.)

- Presence of coughing, aspiration, nasal regurgitation or pain during test swallow.
- Presence of fatigue during consecutive test swallows.
- Mechanical and metabolic factors that may impair swallowing (such as dehydration or the presence of a nasogastric feeding tube).
- Sensory deficits: Loss of touch on the face, lips, and/or oral mucosa; loss of a taste on various areas of the tongue.
- Voice quality: Hoarseness, breathiness, harshness, nasality, and intensity.
- Precision and speed of articulation.
- Respiratory status: Coughing ability, breathing limitations, congestion, respiratory aids.
- Methylene blue aspiration test for a patient with a tracheostomy.

Diagnostic Tests

Indirect laryngoscopy to visualize the anatomy of the thyroid, the function of the vocal cords, and to determine whether there is pooling of secretions and food adjacent to the larynx.

Cineradiography to evaluate all stages of swallowing. (It is particularly useful for evaluation of pharyngeal constriction and the dynamics of airway protection, upper and lower esophageal sphincter function, esophageal motility, morphology of the esophagus, hiatal hernia, and gastro-esophageal reflux.)

Intraluminal esophageal manometry to quantify the velocity of peristalsis and the effectiveness of esophageal contraction and sphincter relaxation.

Other tests may include radiological studies for reflux such as the gastro-esophageal scintiscan. Endoscopy may also be performed to examine local lesions.

Nursing Diagnoses: Actual or Potential

1. Uncompensated swallowing impairment related to muscle weakness or dysfunction of the face, mouth, larynx, pharynx, and/or esophageal sphincters.
2. Potential for aspiration related to swallowing impairment.

3. Self-care deficit: Feeding related to sensory, motor, and/or cognitive deficits.
4. Altered nutritional status: Less than body requirements related to swallowing difficulties.
5. Ineffective individual coping related to swallowing impairment.
6. Anxiety related to loss of swallowing ability, fears of choking.
7. Knowledge deficit related to dysphagia management.

Expected Outcomes: Patient and/or Family

1. The individual follows the correct swallowing sequence for safe oral intake.
2. The individual experiences no aspiration.
3. The individual maintains nutritional status as evidenced by normal skin turgor, stable weight, normal hemoglobin, hematocrit, and serum protein.
4. The individual experiences decreased anxiety and depression as evidenced by verbal statements and/or body language.
5. The individual verbalizes and demonstrates an understanding of dysphagia management.

Planning and Implementation

J. Steefel (1981) has developed a patient classification system to assist in dysphagia program planning (Table 6-1). The management plan should be developed in conjunction with the speech pathologist and be based on the results of the health history, physical assessment, and diagnostic tests. Not every person is a candidate for a dysphagia management program. This is particularly applicable to brain damaged patients who are too cognitively impaired or too agitated to safely participate. Other individuals, because of the severity of their dysphagia, may not be candidates for a feeding program, but may be started on a pre-feeding program that focuses on strengthening the muscles involved in swallowing and increasing the cognitive awareness of the process.

The initial training, involving facial, intraoral, and laryngeal muscle exercises, is usually conducted by the speech pathologist. As the patient progresses, a feeding program is initiated. During the pre-feeding stages the nurse's responsibilities in the program include safety maintenance (close supervision, patient and family in-

TABLE 6-1 Dysphagia Classification System

Classification	Management
Level I. Profound Swallowing Dysfunction	Patient NPO, alternate feeding methods only, pre-feeding activities in oral stimulation and programming
Level II. Marked Swallowing Dysfunction	Alternate feeding methods still primary nutritional source, patient can be fed certain foods but no self feeding, no liquids except in training sessions and via feeding tubes
Level III. Severe Swallowing Dysfunction	Alternate nutritional methods may be discontinued except for fluids, patient should be fairly reliable with prescribed diet though still requires complete supervision; may perform some self-feeding
Level IV. Moderate Swallowing Dysfunction	Patient may still need alternate feeding methods for fluids, patient should be reliable with defined level of food consistency, more difficult foods may be added including clear fluids
Level V. Mild swallowing Dysfunction	Some food restrictions remain, special techniques may still be necessary, patient should no longer require constant supervision
Level VI. Normal Swallowing Function	Competency achieved, patient now completely safe and independent

struction, equipment availability, proper positioning), nutritional maintenance (proper use of prescribed feeding method, intake and weight records), and respiratory management measures to prevent aspiration and congestion (proper positioning, cough and deep breathing exercises, mobilization of secretions, frequent assessments).

Patient and Family Education

After oral feeding is initiated, further coordination is needed between the speech pathologist and the nurse to assure that the plan is followed safely and consistently. Family members need to be included in this plan as well through ongoing explanations of the procedures and frequent opportunities for questions, feedback, and for return demonstrations when appropriate. Posting instructions at the bedside and in the nursing kardex can help to insure the necessary consistency. These instructions should include a list of the foods and fluids allowed and the manner of feeding, positioning guidelines, special equipment needs, special preparation guidelines, and special precautions. Use of a dysphagia flowsheet further assures continuity and facilitates problem resolution by providing an ongoing record of the patient's responses during each feeding session.

The following considerations apply to the nurse and other health team and family members who are working with the patient with dysphagia:

Safety

Maintain a consistent, quiet, distraction-free, unhurried environment at mealtimes. Always have suction equipment available. Place the patient in an upright position with the head flexed forward slightly. Provide posture and head support devices as needed to maintain alignment.

Monitoring

Document patient's weight and nutritional intake on a regular basis. Assess the patient for signs of nutritional deficits and dehydration. Monitor temperature daily and assess respiratory status for signs of aspiration.

Dietary Considerations

Table 6-2 indicates the usual diet progression for the dysphasic patient whose swallowing abilities are continuing to improve.

Procedure for Facilitating Swallowing

The steps for facilitating swallowing are reviewed in Table 6-3.

Psychological Considerations

Avoid using baby food in the dysphagia diet as this can further undermine the patient's self-concept. Reinforce the patient's self-confidence and sense of control by including him/her in all goal setting and program planning. Explore with the patient and family other rewards and socializing opportunities that can help compensate for the loss of eating pleasures. When the patient is anxious, fearful, and/or depressed, provide opportunities for ventilation in a supportive environment; teach relaxation techniques; and refer for counseling when appropriate.

TABLE 6-2 Dysphagia Diet Progression

Diet Level	Foods
1. Dysphagia pureed	Soft boiled eggs, baby food fruits, vegetables, and meats, cottage cheese, mashed potatoes, pudding, custard, thick cereals
2. Dysphagia advanced pureed	Add minced or ground meat, poultry, soft bread
3. Dysphagia mechanical soft	Add soft cooked fruits and vegetables, dry cereals that become soft with milk, soft cakes and sandwiches, potatoes without skin, rice, soft candies
4. Dysphagia soft	Add soft bread and rolls with crusts, scrambled or fried eggs, diced meat and casseroles, all cooked vegetables

Diet Level	Fluids
1. Dysphagia extra thick liquids	Thick soups with added mashed potatoes, juices thickened with pureed fruit or cereal
2. Dysphagia thick liquids	Add less thickening
3. Minimally thickened liquids	Eliminate thickening or add less, may include milk shakes and eggnog
4. Dysphagia clear and other thin liquids	Includes all liquids, also jello and ice cream

Alternatives to Swallowing

For the patient who is not a candidate for a dysphagia program or for one who is suffering nutritional compromises and cannot tolerate a nasogastric tube, alternative feeding methods must be explored. These include surgical procedures such as gastrostomy, jejunostomy, or esophagostomy. (See the medical-surgical reference books for specific information on pre- and post-operative care and how to use feeding tubes and pumps.)

FUTURE IMPLICATIONS

Many dysphagia management programs are ineffective because they don't emphasize the importance of a coordinated team ap-

TABLE 6-3 Swallowing Facilitation Procedure

1. Stimulate mouth opening by lightly stroking it with spoon or applying pressure to chin below lower lip.
2. Place food as far back on tongue as possible without causing gagging, using asepto syringe with tubing attached or glossectomy spoon if necessary.
3. Encourage lip closure with gentle manual pressure.
4. Instruct patient to hold food in mouth briefly to give oral receptors opportunity to trigger reflexes.
5. Encourage swallowing by instructing patient to close lips, hold breath, swallow, and then exhale forcefully.
6. Check for laryngeal elevation and inside of mouth to determine if swallowing occurred.
7. If patient did not swallow, press chin down toward sternum, which elevates larynx and initiates pharyngeal phase; ice sternal notch and briskly rub back of neck near occiput; or stroke neck at each side of trachea.
8. Progress food texture and variety according to patient's tolerance.
9. When fluids are initiated, begin with thick fluids and give to patient on teaspoon.
10. After each feeding, check mouth for retained food and give mouth care.

proach or facilitate such an approach. Other programs fail because of misinterpretation or mismanagement of diagnostic studies. Program failure can also result when team members do not take into account the psychological aspects of swallowing impairments.

When planning a dysphagia management program, consideration must be given to the basic premise that eating and drinking have many meanings for each individual. Psychologically these activities offer opportunities for enhancing feelings of pleasure and self-worth through socializing and sharing. Physically they offer sensory enjoyment and satisfaction, in addition to contributing to health maintenance and survival. The loss of these pleasures and the danger of choking often leaves the person with dysphagia feeling anxious, fearful, and depressed—in addition to being a candidate for fluid and nutritional imbalances. To be successful, a dysphagia management program must address these considerations as well as the procedural and educational components.

REFERENCES

Anderson, B. (1986). Tube feeding: Is diarrhea inevitable? *American Journal of Nursing, 86*(6):704–706.

Brin, M., and Younger, D. (1988). Neurological disorders of aspiration. *Otolarnyolic Clinics of North America, 21*(4):691–699.

DiIorio, C., and Price, M. (1990). Swallowing: An assessment and practice guide. *American Journal of Nursing, 90*(7):38–46.

Emick-Herring, B., and Wood, P. (1990). A team approach to neurologically based swallowing disorders. *Rehabilitation Nursing, 15*(3):126–132.

Hamilton, S. (1987). Self-feeding deficits. In Rehabilitation Nursing Foundation. *Application of Rehabilitation Concepts to Nursing Practice* (2nd ed.). Evanston: Rehabilitation Nursing Foundation.

Logemann, J. (1989). Swallowing disorders and rehabilitation. *Journal of Head Trauma Rehabilitation, 4*(4):1–81.

Logemann, J. (1988). Dysphagia in movement disorders. *Advances in Neurology, 49*:307–316.

Loustaw, A., and Lee, K. (1985). Dealing with the dangers of dysphagia. *Nursing 85, 15*(2):47–50.

Ottenbacher, K. (1985). Reliability of the behavioral assessment scale of oral functions in feeding. *The American Journal of Occupational Therapy, 39*(7):436–440.

Steefel, J. (1981). *Dysphagia rehabilitation for neurologically impaired adults.* Springfield: Charles C. Thomas Publisher.

Sexuality and Disability 7

OBJECTIVES

After completing this chapter, the reader will be able to:

- Discuss the concept of sexuality.
- Describe the sexual response cycle.
- Compare how sexual responses may be affected by spinal cord injury (SCI), multiple sclerosis (MS), amyotrophic lateral sclerosis (ALS), traumatic brain injury (TBI), cerebral vascular accident (CVA), and Parkinson's disease (PD).
- Discuss four psychological concerns that may affect the sexuality of a person with a neurological disability.
- Describe four intervention measures that may facilitate a patient's and partner's sexual readjustment.

INTRODUCTION

Sexuality is a complex concept—an integration of an individual's body image, beliefs, goals, attitudes, relationship to others, and the physiological components of his or her sexual activities. Sexual roles and behavior are further influenced by the person's age, sex, and sociocultural environment. Sustaining a disability can dramatically affect a person's sexuality as it often forces a re-examination of all these aspects of self. For example, many people with disabilities develop a poor self-image as they may feel self-conscious about their physical limitations and unable to fulfill previously defined roles and goals. These feelings can lead to or worsen the depression and anger they may already be feeling at what has happened to them. Interconnected with the poor self-image and depression is often the fear of rejection. The person's negative behavior in anticipation of rejection can result in this fear becoming a reality. Fear of a bowel or bladder accident can further reinforce poor self-image and fear of rejection. Another fear is that sexual activity will cause pain or precipitate medical complications. Guilt about overburdening a partner with extra responsibilities can also affect an intimate relationship.

The able-bodied partner may be experiencing similar feelings—depression and anger over role and lifestyle changes, fear that sexual activity may injure the partner, and guilt over changed feelings toward the partner and over feelings of anger and resentment. Fatigue is another major factor for the able-bodied partner, who may have assumed many additional responsibilities.

Because of these and other physical and psychological issues, the individual with a disability and his/her partner will need a variety of supportive interventions from the rehabilitation nurse and other members of the rehabilitation team to help them achieve a satisfying sexual readjustment. These interventions include offering individual and couple counseling and educational opportunities and facilitating peer group discussions. To provide effective sexual counseling and education, the nurse and other team members must have an understanding of their own sexuality including their sexual values, biases, and problem areas; sensitivity and concern for the patient's and partner's feelings and needs; the ability to listen; and a knowledge of how the psychological and physiological aspects of sexuality are affected by the disability.

EFFECTS OF NEUROLOGICAL IMPAIRMENT ON SEXUAL FUNCTION

Sexual Response Cycle

The excitement phase of the sexual response cycle is initiated when the cortical and subcortical areas of the brain are stimulated by an erotic thought, sight, sound, or smell, or by tactile impulses from other parts of the body. These cortical and subcortical areas then send impulses down the spinal cord. There they trigger responses mediated by the sacral component of the parasympathetic nervous system. The vascular response of genital arterial dilation and vasoconstriction results in penile erection or clitoral enlargement. Other responses occurring during this phase include testes elevation, vaginal and uterine movement, vaginal lubrication, nipple erection, increased muscle tension, and an increase in vital signs. During the plateau phase there is an intensification of all physical responses.

A person with brain damage from disease or trauma may not be able to effectively receive, interpret, and process erotic stimuli to initiate the excitement phase. If a person has spinal cord damage, impulses from the brain may not reach the sacral reflex center to trigger the genital responses. In addition, stimuli below the level of the lesion may not reach the brain for interpretation and processing. However, these stimuli can trigger reflexogenic genital responses via the sacral reflex center without cortical input.

In the orgasm phase there is a release of the buildup of muscle tension and vascular engorgement. The male experiences forceful, expulsive penile contractions, involuntary muscle contractions, emission, and a forceful ejaculation of semen through the external urethral meatus. During ejaculation the bladder sphincter closes, thus preventing retrograde movement of semen into the bladder. The female experiences expulsive uterine contractions, involuntary muscle contractions, and increased vital signs. During the resolution phase there is a return to a relaxed, unstimulated state in both males and females.

If the person with neurological dysfunction has been unable to achieve the physiological responses associated with the excitement and plateau phases of the sexual response cycle, he/she will not be able to achieve the physiological responses associated with orgasm and resolution. (Cardiovascular disease and medications that affect the cardiovascular or nervous system can also impair sexual responses.)

Though neurological damage often interferes with or modifies the physiological responses associated with each phase of the sexual response cycle, persons with neurological disabilities can and do achieve sexual release and pleasure. Those individuals who have impaired genital sensation and function secondary to spinal cord damage can learn alternative methods of initiating the excitement phase and facilitating sexual response. These methods involve amplification of intact sensory areas and using cognitive abilities to maximize the biopsychosexual experience. While persons with brain damage usually do not have impaired genital sensation and function, they are more likely to have increased difficulties achieving sexual release and pleasure, as cortical and subcortical damage can impair cognitive, behavioral, and perceptual abilities. Impairments in these areas can adversely affect the person's judgment, insight, social skills, communication abilities, ability to sustain attention, and integrate sensory stimuli to achieve sexual excitement and fulfillment. In addition to impairing a person's cognitive, behavioral, and perceptual abilities, brain damage can affect libido by damaging the neurohumoral system between the hypothalamus and pituitary gland, which can adversely affect sex hormone production.

Fertility

In addition to affecting libido, the disruption of sex hormone production in some brain injured people can adversely affect fertility in both men and women. Men with other neurological and cardiovascular conditions that have affected erection and ejaculation abilities may also experience fertility problems. Unfortunately there have been no major long-term studies conducted on these groups of men, or on women with various neurological disabilities. The majority of fertility studies in the disabled population have focused on men with SCI. Most of the information obtained from these studies is applicable to men with MS or other types of spinal cord impairment.

A large number of the studies have been conducted over the years at various Veterans Administration Hospitals and they have revealed a high degree of fertility impairment in the subjects studied. There seem to be multiple factors that may contribute to the high infertility rate. One of these factors is the ejaculatory dysfunction. Another factor is erratic temperature control, which may affect the viability of the sperm. The effects of the injury on spermatogenesis are unclear; testicular aspirations and biopsies have resulted in reports of inconsistent microscopic pathological changes in about 50 percent of the cases. Ejaculations produced by injections of papaverine, phentolamine, or prostaglandin E-1; electrical stimulation; or vibromassage have contained millions of motile sperm. In the studies performed, the numbers and quality of the sperm tended to improve with repeated ejaculation, so it remains unclear to what degree testicular function is dependent upon neurotrophic stimulation or whether the changes reported are due to a disuse atrophy.

The fertility in women with spinal cord impairment from injury, tumor, or MS is usually not adversely affected by their conditions. There may be a temporary (weeks to months) cessation of the menstrual cycle directly following the onset of the disability. However, if other health factors are stable, menses resumes and the fertility status remains stable. Women with brain damage that disrupts the neurohormonal cycle are more likely to experience longer term hormonal disruptions with subsequent impairment in their ability to conceive.

OTHER FACTORS THAT CAN AFFECT SEXUAL PERFORMANCE AND PLEASURE

In addition to the psychological factors and neurological effects discussed previously, there are other neurological deficits and environmental factors that can affect the sexual performance and pleasure of a person with a neurological disability and his or her partner.

Neurological Deficits

Mobility Deficits

Most neurological disabilities result in one or more mobility deficits such as weakness, paralysis, spasticity, or rigidity. The extent of the mobility deficit is related to the type and severity of the neurological condition. Mobility limitations determine how sexually active the person can be during a sexual encounter and during the preliminary stages of socializing with and dating potential partners. For many persons, assuming a more passive role physically is difficult and can have a further negative effect on an already poor self-image.

Sensory Deficits

Sensory deficits are another aspect of a neurological disability that can affect sexual pleasure. Many people have decreased sensation in parts of their bodies, including the genital areas, or they experience an uncomfortable hypersensitivity and pain, or they have a combination of all three sensory changes—decreased sensation, hypersensitivity, and pain. Individuals with SCI and MS are most likely to experience decreased sensation, often accompanied by areas of uncomfortable hyperesthesia. Individuals with TBI and CVA are more likely to have problems interpreting sensory changes rather than actually experiencing sensory loss. People with ALS and PD have intact sensation but may experience a great deal of discomfort because of spasticity and mobility limitations.

Sensory deficits can have a major affect on the ability to achieve sexual pleasure. If a person is very uncomfortable or in pain, it is difficult to become involved with and enjoy other activities, including sexual activities. Because cultural programming puts a great deal of emphasis on genital sex, it may be difficult for some people to refocus and relearn other ways of achieving sensual and sexual pleasure.

Fatigue

This is a component of all neurological disabilities. During the first months after the onset of a disability, the individual experiences a high level of fatigue as the body attempts to deal with the physiological insult. This is particularly true when brain damage has occurred from a stroke, tumor, or trauma. Initially they require frequent rest periods throughout the day. In time most people with neurological disabilities are able to resume a more normal sleep/wake schedule, but find that they tire more easily than before their disabilities. However, in certain disabilities fatigue remains an ongoing component and disrupting factor. This is particularly evident with MS, ALS, and CVA. People with these disabilities may not have the energy for many activities, including sexual ones.

Effects Related to Each Disability

Table 7-1 indicates the neurological deficits encountered in each disability which may affect sexual performance and pleasure.

Environmental Factors

Lack of privacy is a major impediment to sexual exploration and pleasure. Most hospitals and rehabilitation centers do not have adequate facilities to provide private space for individual patients. Even after a person is discharged to home, lack of privacy often continues to be a complicating factor if additional assistance is re-

TABLE 7-1 Disability-related Factors Affecting Sexual Performance

Disability	Factors Affecting Sexual Performance
Spinal Cord Injury	Erection and ejaculation dysfunction in males Impaired fertility in males Decreased vaginal lubrication in females Mobility and sensory deficits Bowel and bladder incontinence
Multiple Sclerosis	Fatigue and decreased physical endurance Erection and ejaculation dysfunction in males Impaired fertility in males Decreased vaginal lubrication in females Mobility and sensory deficits Bladder dysfunction
Amyotrophic Lateral Sclerosis	Fatigue and decreased physical endurance Erection and ejaculation dysfunction in males in later stages of disease Impaired fertility in males in later stages of disease Decreased vaginal lubrication in females in later stages of disease Mobility deficits
Cerebral Vascular Accident	Fatigue and decreased physical endurance Mobility and sensory deficits Communication deficits Perceptual and visual deficits Cognitive and behavioral deficits Erection and ejaculation dysfunction in males Decreased vaginal lubrication in females and changes in menstrual pattern
Traumatic Brain Injury	Cognitive and behavioral deficits Perceptual and visual deficits Communication deficits Mobility and sensory deficits depending on location and extent of brain damage
Parkinson's Disease	Erection and ejaculation dysfunction in males Decreased vaginal lubrication in females Mobility deficits Communication deficits Cognitive deficits

quired for daily care and if accessibility problems limit the private rooms available.

Accessibility outside of the home can also impact on the individual's social life and sexual relationships. This applies particularly to the person who is not currently living with a partner. He or she may become increasingly isolated from outside contacts and potential partners.

NURSING INTERVENTIONS

Assessment

Health History

- Previous methods of coping and current effectiveness.
- History of psychological problems.
- Interpersonal skills and behavior.
- Current self-image.
- Age.
- Changes in vocational and socioeconomic status and family role.
- Presence and status of intimate relationships.
- Partner's perception of the relationship and future possibilities.
- Cultural and religious beliefs in relation to sex.
- Comfort in talking about sexual issues.
- Concerns and goals regarding sexual issues and education.
- Previous knowledge about sexuality.
- Health/sexual problems prior to the disability.

Physical Assessment

- Type of disability.
- Physical abilities and limitations, including balance and endurance.
- Presence of spasticity and effect on various positions.
- Presence (or absence) of erections and effective stimuli.
- Type and location of sensory deficits.
- Presence and type of communication deficits.
- Bowel and bladder problems and current management.
- Presence of genital lesions or other abnormalities.

Diagnostic Tests

(Certain tests may be performed depending on the individual's presenting problem.)

- Fertility workup.
- Nocturnal penile tumescence study (NPT) to determine if the erection dysfunction is organic or psychogenic.

Nursing Diagnoses: Actual or Potential

1. Sexual dysfunction related to motor, sensory, and/or cognitive deficits, role changes, self-concept disturbance, lack of privacy, reduced activity tolerance, knowledge deficit.
2. Disturbance in self-concept related to changes in body image and in sexual role and abilities.
3. A reactive depression related to changes and/or losses of body functions, change in lifestyle, role change, negative self-concept.
4. Anxiety related to threat to self-concept, sexual functioning and interaction patterns; unmet needs.
5. Knowledge deficit related to lack of education and sexual experience since the disability.

Expected Outcomes: Patient and/or Partner

1. The individual verbalizes perception of himself/herself as a sexual being.
2. The individual discusses sexual issues and concerns.
3. The individual reports a satisfying sexual relationship.
4. The individual experiences decreased anxiety as evidenced by verbal statements and/or body language.
5. The individual verbalizes and demonstrates an understanding of disability-related changes in sexual functioning, pleasuring techniques, birth control methods, AIDS and venereal disease preventive measures appropriately.

Planning and Implementation

Frequently in society and in rehabilitation settings there is too much emphasis placed on physical aspects of sex and too little attention is given to the larger and more important issues involving a person's sexuality. Sustaining a disability can have a profound effect on all elements of sexuality. Therefore, sexuality programs must be initiated that have this broader focus. Each patient needs a spectrum of support options to assist him or her in regaining self confidence and improving self-image and communication skills. Professional collaboration with the patient in addressing concerns and setting goals is essential. An interdisciplinary approach is needed to accomplish these goals through the avenues of individual and couple counseling, peer counseling, and therapeutic groups/classes that provide opportunities for sharing, supporting, developing interpersonal and communication skills, and for learning about the various aspects of sexuality and approaches for achieving sexual pleasure.

Self Assessment

Prior to beginning a sexual counseling and education plan, it is important for the nurse to perform an honest self assessment of his or her own sexuality, biases, values and discomforts to avoid imposing these on the patient. An awareness of and respect for one's limitations is an integral part of such an assessment. Not all nurses are comfortable addressing sexuality issues in themselves or in others. Using a cognitive self therapy approach may be helpful in dealing with and overcoming some of the discomfort and nontherapeutic attitudes. The focus of this approach is to identify a particular issue and the thoughts and feelings evoked by the issue. If there is a desire to change certain thoughts and feelings, the individual examines alternative ways of responding and develops a plan that works toward the integration of preferable alternatives.

Counseling

Sexual counseling is one of the primary methods used to facilitate a healthy psychosexual readjustment in the person with a disability. Table 7-2 highlights some of the elements involved in successful interviewing and sexual counseling. Under certain circumstances the nurse is advised to initiate a referral to a therapist rather than attempting to handle the counseling and sexual education independently. These circumstances include when the patient and partner have a long history of pre-disability problems; when the nurse lacks resources, comfort, or training in the area or does not have adequate time for counseling; and when the patient and/or partner show evidence of severe depression or substance abuse problems.

Therapeutic and Educational Groups

Another form of intervention to facilitate psychosexual adjustment is with therapeutic groups. Such groups provide the patients

TABLE 7-2 Counseling Techniques

1. Conduct all interviewing and counseling in a private setting and strive to maintain a relaxed, unhurried atmosphere.
2. Determine what the patient's and partner's priorities are (refer to assessment).
3. Determine what sexuality means to each person and work within this moral and religious context.
4. Use common terminology and avoid medical and professional terms.
5. Maintain eye contact, continuous reassurance, and a matter-of-fact approach to help establish comfort.
6. Be a model of openness and comfort.
7. Be aware of personal biases and do not attempt to impose these on the patient (see self-assessment).
8. In beginning the discussion, start with the least sensitive topics.
9. Use nondirective techniques and avoid using loaded or leading questions.
10. Use open-ended questions to give the person a variety of answers to choose from depending on his or her comfort level.

and partners with opportunities for self-exploration, understanding their relationship with others, enhancing a sense of control and confidence, developing social and communication skills, and sharing. Groups also offer a forum for presenting information related to the concerns of the participants. Learning is facilitated when the leaders clarify ideas that are unclear, provide positive feedback, and encourage the participants to discover answers to their own questions.

The requirements for nurses to be successful group leaders/teachers are similar to those for effective counselors. They must be aware of and comfortable with their own sexuality, knowledgeable about the subject, comfortable in its presentation, and knowledgeable about how to most effectively teach the patients. They must also be tolerant and accepting of a variety of sexual behaviors and feelings. Their approaches must be open, honest, and flexible.

Cofacilitation of groups/classes by a nurse and another health team member such as a psychologist or social worker can be extremely beneficial. These two groups of health professionals have knowledge and skills in counseling and group work that can be integrated with the knowledge and skills of the nurses to maximize the participant's experience.

The following sections provide information on managing specific concerns and problems that the patients may encounter. Prior to presenting information on sexuality and on specific issues, the leader/teacher needs to determine the learning needs and knowledge levels of the participants in the group based on the results of the individual assessments. The initial presentation of information can usually be handled satisfactorily in a class setting. The patient and partner must also be provided with opportunities to deal with individual concerns in a private setting.

Management Options for Erectile and Ejaculatory Dysfunction

For the man who is experiencing erectile dysfunction as a result of his disability, penile prostheses are available. The three main types include the semi-rigid silicone rods, which give a permanent semi-erect penis, flexible silicone rods which can be bent into position for intercourse, and the inflatable prosthesis, which can be maximally inflated to achieve a full erection when desired. Psychological counseling and a complete physical assessment are required to determine if the man is an appropriate candidate for a prosthesis and, if so, to determine which type would most effectively meet his needs.

Another option for managing erectile dysfunction is with the use of vacuum tumescence such as the Erecaid System. This system is composed of a plastic cylinder, tubing, a vacuum hand pump, and rubber constriction/retention bands. A vacuum is produced in the cylinder which then draws blood into the corpora of the penis, producing engorgement and rigidity. A structured patient education program and adequate practice are necessary before the device is issued.

For the man with ejaculatory dysfunction there are three methods under investigation for triggering ejaculation. These methods include electrical stimulation, chemical stimulation with injections of papaverine, phentolamine, or prostaglandin E-1, and vibrator stimulation. At this time no consistently successful method has been discovered. However, vibromassage appears to be the safest and most readily available method.

Birth Control

Because fertility is not affected in many women with disabilities, methods of birth control need to be reviewed. The birth control pill is probably the most widely discussed and debated method of birth control among members of the medical community. Except for sterilization it is the most effective method and is easy to use. However, studies reveal that pills with a high estrogen content cause a significant increase in the risk of blood clots in the able-bodied population. Unfortunately, no studies of the clot risk factor have been conducted with disabled women, but it is likely increased, as most of these women are already facing an increased clotting risk secondary to immobility. Other side effects to consider with progesterone/based birth control pills are weight gain and the depression some women experience, which may be magnified for the disabled women going through major lifestyle adjustments.

The safest methods of nonpermanent birth control are the diaphragm, sponge, and a condom-foam combination. While the diaphragm and sponge are relatively safe and effective, they do require manual dexterity for proper insertion. The rhythm method is preferred by some couples. However, this is usually less effective than other methods and if pregnancy is a definite health hazard, this would not be the most effective choice.

Pregnancy

The woman with a disability who does want children should seek out an obstetrician familiar with her disability. While her pregnancy may be similar to that of a woman without a disability, she still will need certain special considerations. Many of the potential problems associated with pregnancy may be more likely to occur and may be more severe in the disabled woman. These include phlebitis, blood pressure changes, urinary tract infections, and constipation. Therefore, the individual needs instructions on how to prevent and manage these problems. She will also need to be aware of special problems related to her specific disability. For example, the woman with a SCI above T6 may experience autonomic hyper-reflexia during labor and delivery and would require close monitoring and supervision. Becoming pregnant creates a high risk situation for any disabled woman with severe pre-existing medical problems.

Sexual Arousal Techniques

For the person with compromised genital sensation, other techniques need to be explored to enable him or her to achieve sexual arousal and release. The primary methods involve using various forms of sensory amplification. To do this a person maximizes responsiveness to all the sensory avenues that are intact. This usually includes visual, auditory, and olfactory stimulation, as well as tactile stimulation of any sensory intact areas of the body. These physical stimuli, accompanied by sexual fantasies and other psychological stimuli, can increase the individual's level of sexual excitement to the point of orgasm. Those people who do not reach orgasm may still experience some of the physiological changes associated with the orgasm and resolution phases of the sexual response cycle. For the person with brain damage, the techniques to achieve sexual arousal will depend on the type and extent of his/her cognitive and behavioral deficits.

Communication

Open communication between partners is an essential element of all aspects of sexual interaction. Each partner needs to share what pleases and what does not in a physical sense. Equally important is the sharing and communicating of feelings of love, affection, and commitment. When one partner has a communication deficit, the couple may need guidance in developing alternative methods to communicate preferences and feelings.

Timing and Environment

As with any couple the timing of sexual activities and the environmental cues can greatly enhance or detract from the experiences. Since fatigue is a major factor for many people with disabilities and for their partners, and optimum time must be selected when both individuals are rested and not rushed. Also, for those individuals who have problems with spasticity, an optimum time may be when the spasms are reduced, such as after a warm shower or after receiving antispasticity medication. The optimum environment provides quiet, privacy, and other forms of sensory input that are sexually stimulating for the couple.

Personal Care

Because appearance has a major effect on how people view themselves and how others view them, patients should be instructed on how to most effectively manage hygiene and grooming tasks in relation to their disability-related limitations. Another consideration that may pose a problem is when the nondisabled partner is helping the disabled individual with his or her bowel and bladder routines.

It may be difficult for him/her to have sexual feelings toward that person. It may be better in these cases for a visiting nurse or aide to handle such matters.

Positioning

Finding a position that will be comfortable, limit spasticity, and compensate for lack of mobility can be difficult. Many couples prefer a face to face sidelying position, as this allows them multiple sources of stimulation without placing either partner in a strained or dependent position. Some disabled individuals may achieve more functional movement by taking advantage of spasms. Others may experience more limitations because of them. Each couple needs to explore and find what is pleasing and acceptable to them. A waterbed is preferred by many, as it is more comfortable than a standard mattress and may maximize mobility for the disabled partner.

Bowel and Bladder

If a woman has an indwelling catheter, it is often easiest to leave it in but taped to the abdomen so it will not be pulled out. A man with a catheter can fold it back over the erect penis or allow enough slack for erection. A condom can then be applied. Women and men without catheters may prefer to limit fluid intake and to empty the bladder prior to intercourse. The possibility of a bowel accident occurring during sexual activity is a major concern for many persons with disabilities. Pre-planning is the best insurance to avoid having intercourse near the bowel routine time or when the routine has been greatly disrupted.

AIDS and Venereal Disease Prevention

Preventing these diseases is a national concern for all population groups that are sexually active. Education on causes, symptoms, and preventive measures is applicable to both the able-bodied and disabled community.

FUTURE IMPLICATIONS

With the exception of men with spinal cord injuries the subject of sexuality and disability has not been given sufficient attention from either a psychosocial or physiological perspective in the rehabilitation literature. Additional studies are needed to increase understanding of these perspectives in relation to each disability and to identify the most effective methods to assist the individual in adjusting to disability-related changes in his/her sexual abilities and self-concept.

REFERENCES

Blackerby, W. (1990). Sexualtiy and head injury. *Journal of Head Trauma Rehabilitation, 5*(2):1–82.

Burgener, S., and Logan, G. (1989). Sexuality concerns of the post stroke patient. *Rehabilitation Nursing, 14*(4):178–181, 195.

Emick, H. (1985). Sexual changes in patients and partners following stroke. *Rehabilitation Nursing, 10*(2):28–30.

Hamilton, S. (1987). Sexuality and disability. In Rehabilitation Nursing Foundation. *Application of Rehabilitation Concepts to Nursing Practice.* Evanston: Rehabilitation Nursing Foundation, pp. 189–192.

Hanak, M. (1986). *Patient and family education.* New York: Springer Publishing Company.

Hogan, R. (1985). *Human sexuality: A nursing perspective.* Norwalk: Appleton-Century-Crofts.

Lloyd, E., Toth, L., and Perkash, I. (1989). Vacuum tumescence: An option for spinal cord injured males with erectile dysfunction. *SCI Nursing, 6*(2):25–28.

Masters, W., Johnson, V., and Kolodny, R. (1986). *Masters and Johnson on sex and human loving.* Boston: Little, Brown, and Company.

McCormick, G., Reffer, D., and Thompson, M. (1986). Coital positioning for stroke afflicted couples. *Rehabilitation Nursing, 11*(2):17–19.

Monga, T., Lawson, J., and Inglis, I. (1986). Sexual dysfunction in stroke patients. *Archives of Physical Medicine and Rehabilitation, 67*:19–22.

Poorman, S. (1988). *Human sexuality and the nursing process.* Norwalk: Appleton and Lange.

Price, J. (1985). Promoting sexual wellness in head-injured patients. *Rehabilitation Nursing, 10*(6):12–13.

Steinke, E., and Bergen, M. (1986). Sexuality and aging. *Journal of Gerontological Nursing, 12*(6):6–10.

White, E. (1986). Appraising the need for altered sexuality information. *Rehabilitation Nursing, 11*(3):6–9.

Williams, L. (1989). Pharmacologic erection programs: Treatment option for erectile dysfunction. *Rehabilitation Nursing, 14*(5):264–268.

Nursing Management of Specific Neurological Disabilities

PART

III

Traumatic Brain Injury Management

8

OBJECTIVES

After completing this chapter, the reader will be able to:

- Describe the basic pathophysiology of brain injury.
- Compare and contrast focal and diffuse brain injuries.
- Describe five potential neurological complications following brain injury and their manifestations.
- Describe the cognitive processes frequently disrupted with traumatic brain injury (TBI) and the related manifestations of cognitive impairment.
- Describe treatment measures for four categories of cognitive dysfunction.
- Discuss the manifestations of behavioral dysfunction and the factors that may contribute to it.
- Describe the treatment approaches for four categories of behavioral dysfunction.
- Discuss the type of family problems that frequently develop after TBI and appropriate management recommendations.

INTRODUCTION

Approximately 44,000 people per year survive severe TBI with moderate to severe neurobehavioral and physical sequelae. The highest incidence of TBI is found in the 15- to 24-year-old age group and in those from 65 to 75 years. Males are two to three times more likely to be injured than females. It has also been noted that TBI occurs with greater frequency among minority and lower socioeconomic groups. About one half of all TBI's are caused by motor vehicle accidents. The other 50% are primarily the result of falls and assaults. Individuals who are at highest risk for sustaining TBI's are those who have consumed alcohol prior to driving a motor vehicle, those who have had previous head injuries, or those who have psychiatric illnesses.

The individual with a TBI presents the nurses and the entire rehabilitation team with a unique challenge. The team must be prepared to identify and treat a wide range of physical, cognitive, and behavioral deficits resulting from the brain injury, as the pattern of deficits varies greatly from one injured individual to the next. In addition, each team member needs to integrate their skills and knowledge with other team members in a nondiscipline-specific manner. The major focus of TBI rehabilitation is to assist the injured individual in restructuring, integrating, and maximizing cognitive, behavioral, and physical abilities. Therefore, it is crucial that the team members provide a well-coordinated, structured, and integrated program to assure the highest probability of successfully achieving these goals.

PATHOPHYSIOLOGY

Brain damage following trauma results from two mechanisms—primary and secondary injury. The ultimate mortality and morbidity of TBI relates to a combination of effects from these pathological processes.

Primary Injuries

Primary injury is caused by the impact of the trauma. When the dura remains intact, the injury is referred to as a closed or blunt trauma. Penetration of the dura results in exposure of the cranial contents to the environment and is referred to as an open or penetrating trauma. Primary injuries are further classified as focal or diffuse injuries.

A contusion is the most common form of focal injury. The force of the impact produces the contusion at the point the brain is in contact with the skull (coup injury). A rebound effect usually produces another contusion on the opposite side of the brain (coup contre-coup injury). In addition to causing the contusion, the force of impact injures blood vessels in the vicinity, which in turn produces subdural and intracerebral hematomas and epidural hemorrhage. The severity of injury is associated with the amount of energy transmitted by the skull to the underlying brain tissue. Also, the smaller the area of impact the greater the severity of injury in that area because the force is concentrated. Penetrating injuries are another type of focal injury. Brain damage occurs along the path of the bullet or sharp projectile.

With diffuse injuries, rapid acceleration, deceleration, and rotation forces cause shearing, tearing, and/or stretching of the nerve fibers in the brain with subsequent blood vessel and axonal damage. Diffuse axonal injuries (DAI) account for the greatest number of severely disabled TBI survivors due to the extensive disruption of neural connections to all areas of the brain.

Secondary Injury Processes

With secondary injury a combination of interrelated events occurs, which can extend the destruction caused by the primary injury. Vasogenic edema occurs as a result of the disruption of the blood brain barrier. The edema and the related elevated intracranial pressure (ICP) compromise the arterial blood flow and venous return, leading to hypoxia and acidosis. These conditions cause disrupted cell metabolism and increased vasodilation. The combination of vascular and metabolic disturbances cause a further increase in edema and ICP leading to a self-perpetuating cycle of increasing hypoxia and cell death. Other factors that can elevate ICP and cause further brain damage include hematomas, depressed skull fractures, pain, elevated temperature, and venous obstruction.

Systemic factors such as respiratory failure and hypoxia, cardiac arrest, blood loss, hypotension, and emboli may also contribute to secondary brain injury.

Severity Classifications

The Glasgow Coma Scale (GCS) is one of the tools used to define the severity of brain injury and predict its outcome. This scale re-

TABLE 8-1 Glasgow Coma Scale

Eyes	Open	Spontaneously	4
		To verbal command	3
		To pain	2
	No response		1
Best motor response	To verbal command	Obeys	6
	To painful stimulus	Localizes pain	5
		Flexion-withdrawal	4
		Flexion-abnormal (decerebrate rigidity)	3
		Extension (decerebrate rigidity)	2
		No response	1
Best verbal response		Oriented and converses	5
		Disoriented and converses	4
		Inappropriate words	3
		Incomprehensible sounds	2
		No response	1
Total			3-15

lates consciousness to motor response, verbal response, and eye opening (Table 8-1). Usually a combination of parameters is used to define the severity of injury (Uomoto, 1990):

- Mild injury—pretrauma amnesia of 10 to 60 minutes, coma of 0 to 2 hours, and a GCS score of 12 to 15.
- Moderate injury—pretrauma amnesia of 1 to 24 hours, coma of 1 to 6 hours, and a GCS score of 9 to 11.
- Severe injury—pretrauma amnesia of 1 to 7 days, coma of more than 6 hours, and a GCS score of 3 to 8.

Recovery and Outcome

Nervous system recovery involves neurophysiological/neuroanatomical, and behavioral/functional reorganization. Four mechanisms of recovery may operate: resolution of temporary factors, neuronal regeneration, denervation supersensitivity, and functional substitution. In spontaneous early recovery (first days to weeks following injury) re-establishment of uninjured neural systems may occur as a result of resolution of secondary injury processes. This type of recovery is attributed to the following physiological events: Blood and edema are reabsorbed; blood flow returns to normal; electrolyte and neurotransmitter balance is re-established.

Long-term recovery (weeks to months following injury) may involve a process of regeneration of neural elements manifested by axonal growth. In this process axons sprout from the end of damaged axons over a period of weeks to months and from the sides of undamaged axons (collateralization) over a period of days to weeks. The importance of axonal sprouting is unclear for a number of reasons: fiber sprouting may be age dependent, occurring most readily in infancy; it has only been demonstrated over short distances and primarily in nonmammal species; and the possibility of consistent functional improvement has not been demonstrated. With denervation supersensitivity there is postsynaptic receptor site proliferation and increased sensitivity to neurotransmitter agents in denervated neurons.

Long-term recovery may also involve the process of functional substitution. In this process axons that performed a comparable or subservient function prior to injury take over the function of damaged fibers in the area. Also, fibers not initially involved with a particular function take on the new role through a training program. At this time the degree to which functional substitution occurs in TBI rehabilitation is unclear.

Factors Influencing Recovery

Factors that influence recovery include the site of injury, the extent and magnitude of nervous system damage, the time since onset, the rate of improvement immediately following injury, and the presence of complications and associated injuries. Patient characteristics influencing recovery include age, developmental level, premorbid level of function and physical condition, history of drug abuse, the presence of drugs and alcohol at the time of injury, socioeconomic status, interpersonal resources, and medical risk factors. Of these, the most significant outcome predictors are the severity and extent of injury and the initial rate of improvement.

The time required for outcome to become stable has not been fully established. However, the general consensus is that an individual's overall levels of disability and dependence become stabilized within one year of injury, with the most progress evident in the first 3 to 6 months. The Glasgow Outcome Scale and its modified version, the Disability Rating Scale, are tools used to describe and evaluate outcome. Each consists of categories related to severity of disability. Social, physical, and cognitive parameters are used to determine an individual's category.

Neurological Complications

Hydrocephalus resulting from ventricular obstruction occurs in up to 40% of individuals with severe TBI. It usually begins to appear within 2 weeks of injury. The primary method of management is with shunt insertion.

Post traumatic epilepsy is common after severe TBI. It occurs in 15 to 20% of persons during the acute phase following injury. Up to 50% of individuals with TBI will develop a late onset seizure disorder up to one to 2 years after injury. Persons at risk for developing a seizure disorder include those who have sustained an open head injury, a depressed skull fracture and/or a brain hematoma, and those who have experienced an early seizure (one week post injury). Initial treatment for individuals at high risk for seizure is the administration of parenteral phenytoin (Dilantin) or phenobarbital. Because these drugs can impair cognitive performance, carbamazepine (Tegretol) or valproic acid (Depakene) are preferred when oral administration is feasible. If an individual is seizure-free for one year he/she should be weaned off of all anti-seizure medications.

Hypothalamic and pituitary injuries can result in diabetes insipidus (DI) or the syndrome of inappropriate antidiuretic hormone secretion. Both disorders are managed acutely by controlling fluid and electrolyte intake and by monitoring serum electrolytes and osmolality. Persistence of late onset DI is frequently managed with vasopressin (Pitressin) or desmopressin (DDAVP). Pituitary damage may also result in panhypopituitarism or in a selective loss of thyrotropin, adrenocorticotropic hormone, or gonadal stimulating hormones. Replacement therapy and close monitoring are the primary management objectives.

Elevated ICP is managed with measures that act on cerebral blood flow, edema, and metabolic activity. These measures include hyperosmolytic diuretics, steroids, barbiturates, fluid restriction, hyperventilation, and hypothermia. Preventive measures to avoid vascular obstruction include careful positioning with the head of the bed elevated 15 to 30 degrees, avoidance of prone lying, neck flexion, and extreme hip flexion, and avoidance of the valsalva maneuver through bowel management measures and patient instructions, when feasible.

Hematomas usually require surgical evacuation. Preventing recurrent bleeding remains an ongoing concern. Infection prevention is also an ongoing concern. Individuals at particular risk for infection are those with open head injuries and those requiring surgical intervention.

Cognitive Dysfunction

The following cognitive processes are frequently disrupted after a diffuse brain injury involving the frontal and temporal lobes: attention, memory, abstract reasoning, generalization, concept formation, problem solving, and executive function. Disruption of these processes leads to a breakdown in the ability to filter out irrelevant background stimuli, to learn new information, to comprehend the essence of what is happening in a specific situation or conversation, to apply old solutions to new situations, to generate different solutions for specific problems, or to self-direct and follow through with a plan. The manifestations of cognitive impairment are identified on page 119. While some of these manifestations of cognitive dysfunction are obvious, others may not be as overt. To avoid misunderstandings and improper treatment, it is essential that each individual with TBI receive a comprehensive, systematic interdisciplinary evaluation.

In addition to this indepth evaluation, certain tools are used to provide interdisciplinary documentation for observations of cognitive progress and as a guide for interventions. One of the most frequently used tools is the Rancho Los Amigos Levels of Cognitive Functioning (Table 8-2).

Behavioral Dysfunction

Diffuse brain injury often results in the following deficits in behavioral function: Inability to structure and/or modify emotional reactions, inability to deal appropriately and flexibly with ongoing environmental stimuli and events, and inability to affect and maintain appropriate relationship between the self and the environment.

TABLE 8-2 Rancho Los Amigos Scale of Cognitive Levels and Expected Behavior

Level I	No Response	Unresponsive to all stimuli
Level II	Generalized Response	Inconsistent, nonpurposeful, non-specific reactions to stimuli. Responds to pain, but response may be delayed.
Level III	Localized Response	Inconsistent reaction directly related to type of stimulus presented. Responds to some commands. May respond to discomfort.
Level IV	Confused, Agitated Response	Disoriented and unaware of present events with frequent bizarre and inappropriate behavior. Attention span is short and ability to process information is impaired.
Level V	Confused Inappropriate Nonagitated Response	Nonpurposeful random or fragmented responses when task complexity exceeds abilities. Patient appears alert and responds to simple commands. Performs previously learned tasks but is unable to learn new ones.
Level VI	Confused Appropriate Response	Behavior is goal directed. Responses are appropriate to the situation with incorrect responses due to memory difficulties.
Level VII	Automatic Appropriate Response	Correct routine responses which are robotlike. Appears oriented to setting, but insight, judgment and problem-solving are poor.
Level VIII	Purposeful Appropriate Response	Correct responding, carryover of new learning. No required supervision, poor tolerance for stress, and some abstract reasoning difficulties.

Reprinted with permission from Rancho Los Amigos, Downey, CA.

Manifestations of these behavioral disorders are identified on pages 119–120.

Behavior disorders are classified as positive (disorders that actively interfere with the rehabilitation process) and negative (disorders of drive and motivation). Positive behavior disorders are categorized as aggressive, sexual, or attention seeking. Negative behavior disorders are categorized primarily as problems with arousal. Secondary behavior disturbances frequently encountered in the individual with TBI include denial, depression, and dependence on others.

The site of the lesion is the most significant determinant of the presence and severity of behavioral dysfunction. Frontal lobe injuries are characterized by decreased drive, apathy, social disinhibition, emotional lability, flat affect, egocentricity, childishness, lack of self-esteem, lack of goal-directed behavior, and lack of insight. Temporal lobe injuries are characterized by disinhibition and aggression. Hypothalamic and basilar branch injuries are characterized by sluggishness, mood swings, irritability, sleep disturbances, and appetite irregularities. Premorbid conditions such as maladaptive behavior patterns and familiar psychiatric instability can exacerbate lesion-based behavior disorders, as can adjustment factors such as anxiety, depression, social isolation, and impaired social relationships.

NURSING INTERVENTIONS

Assessment

Health History

- Mechanism of injury, time since injury, and associated injuries.
- History of loss of consciousness and duration.
- Systems review indicating problems experienced since injury.
- Pre-existing conditions or disease.
- Current medications
- Known allergies
- Personal history including diet, sleep, smoking, and exercise patterns and psychosocial status.

Physical Assessment Findings

Vital sign instability, presence of headache, nausea, vomiting.

Cognitive dysfunction evidenced by impaired arousal; confusion; impaired ability to concentrate and maintain attention; impaired memory; impaired abstract thinking and reasoning; impaired generalization, concept formation, and planning abilities; executive function deficits; impaired judgment.

Communication deficits evidenced by impaired written and verbal comprehension and output (confabulation, circumlocution, perseveration, anomia, confused speech, apraxia, aphasia).

Behavior disturbances evidenced by dependency and reduced initiation, impulsivity and disinhibition, restlessness and irritability, reduced tolerance to stress, increased emotional lability, aggression, egocentricity and social inappropriateness, withdrawal, depression, and apathy.

Motor dysfunction evidenced by paresis, paralysis, spasticity, ataxia, impaired balance, decreased endurance, pathological reflexes.

Impaired visual spatial orientation evidenced by cortical blindness and visual field deficits.

Sensory perceptual deficits evidenced by impaired position sense and spatial judgment; impaired temperature, pain, and touch awareness; tactile defensiveness; apraxias; agnosias.

Cranial nerve dysfunction evidenced by dysphagia, diplopia, dysarthria, impaired taste and smell, hearing loss.

Diagnostic Tests

Computed tomography (CT scan) to detect hydrocephalus, brain swelling, intracranial hematomas, or infarction.

Magnetic resonance imaging (MRI) to detect abnormalities in the brain.

Positron emission tomography (PET scan) to demonstrate chemical activity in the brain and to show the extent of tissue damage.

Electroencephalogram (EEG) to provide information on the severity, location, and extent of brain damage.

Multimodality evoked potentials (MEPs) to detect and localize visual, auditory, and somatosensory deficits.

Echoencephalography to detect shift of cerebral midline structures.

Skull films to reveal cranium fractures.

Nursing Diagnoses: Actual or Potential

1. Altered thought processes related to attention, memory, abstraction, reasoning, concept formation, generalization, problem solving, and executive function deficits.
2. Impaired physical mobility related to paresis, spasticity, ataxia, impaired balance, decreased endurance.
3. Impaired communication related to aphasia, dysarthria, dyslexia, dysgraphia.
4. Sensory perceptual alterations: visual, auditory, kinesthetic,

tactile related to altered sensory reception, transmission and/
or integration.

5. Self-care deficits: feeding, bathing/hygiene, dressing/groom-
   ing, toileting related to sensory, motor, and cognitive deficits;
   fatigue, depression.
6. Potential for injury related to sensory, motor, cognitive deficits, and/or seizure activity.
7. Activity intolerance related to deconditioning and/or motor
   deficits.
8. Respiratory dysfunction: Pulmonary congestion and atelectasis related to immobility; aspiration related to dysphagia.
9. Impaired skin integrity related to immobility, mechanical
   factors, altered nutritional status, sensory and cognitive
   deficits.
10. Altered bowel elimination: Incontinence related to cognitive
    deficits, constipation or diarrhea related to tube feedings
    and/or medication side effects.
11. Altered nutritional status: Less than body requirements re-
    lated to chewing/swallowing difficulties, inability to feed
    self.
12. Uncompensated swallowing impairment related to neurologi-
    cal dysfunction.
13. Altered urinary elimination: Incontinence related to cognitive
    and motor deficits.
14. Sexual dysfunction related to biopsychosocial alteration of
    sexuality, absence of role models, lack of privacy, lack of
    knowledge.
15. Social isolation related to cognitive, sensory, and motor defi-
    cits; self-concept disturbances.
16. Disturbance in self-concept: Body image, self-esteem.
17. Anxiety related to threat to self-concept, role functioning and
    interaction patterns; unmet needs.
18. Ineffective individual or family coping related to inadequate
    information, inadequate support, multiple life changes.
19. Knowledge deficit related to TBI management.

Expected Outcomes: Patient and/or Family

1. The individual progresses to a higher level of cognitive functioning.

2. The individual maintains functional alignment and sustains no complications of immobility.
3. The individual employs an effective method of communication to convey thoughts and needs.
4. The individual uses correct techniques to facilitate mobility and to compensate for motor and sensory deficits.
5. The individual re-establishes role functions and socialization patterns and engages in self-care activities consistent with cognitive, motor, and sensory deficits, and tolerance level.
6. The individual remains free of injury.
7. The individual's lungs remain clear.
8. The individual's skin remains intact.
9. The individual is free of urinary and bowel complications.
10. The individual's bowel and bladder patterns are stabilized.
11. The individual maintains nutritional status as evidenced by stable weight and normal hematocrit, hemoglobin, and serum protein.
12. The individual verbalizes perception of himself/herself as a sexual being in a manner consistent with cognitive status.
13. The individual experiences decreased anxiety and improved self-concept as evidenced by verbal statements and/or body language.
14. The individual verbalizes and demonstrates an understanding of TBI management.

Planning and Implementation

(Include the family, significant other, and/or caregiver in the teaching interventions.)

Systemic Management

Refer to the following pages for specific management information: dysphagia pages 81–92; uninhibited bladder pages 51–68; uninhibited bowel pages 69–70; skin care pages 146–148; respiratory care pages 144–145.

There are special nutritional considerations for the patient with TBI as the injury can produce dramatic increases in basal metabolism, which leads to weight loss, low serum albumin levels, and a negative nitrogen balance. Steroid administration further exacerbates these conditions.

Monitor the patient's weight, serum albumin and nitrogen levels and hemoglobin and hematocrit. Work with the nutritionist to provide the patient with a high calorie, high protein diet individualized to meet his/her nutrient needs.

Some of the motor disorders associated with TBI present a special management challenge. Ataxia is particularly difficult to treat. Selective splinting and a weighted walker may be beneficial. Levodopa (L-Dopa), and propanolol (Inderal) have been used to treat both the ataxia and tremors associated with TBI. Success is variable with these medications and other drug interventions are under investigation. Weakness is treated with active assistive range of motion and progressive assistive exercises. Slowed motor response is another common disorder which appears to be related to a central processing delay rather than a specific motor deficit. There is no common treatment approach that has been beneficial with this motor processing problem. Managing spasticity also presents special difficulties as the standard antispastic drugs such as diazepam (Valium), baclofen (Lioresal) and dantrolene (Dantrium) further impair cognitive abilities. Therefore, other types of intervention such as special positioning and phenol nerve blocks are preferable.

Work with the physical and occupational therapists to maintain a consistent and individualized program of exercises and positioning to minimize the patient's motor deficits. Administer medications as prescribed. Observe and record the patient's response. Take precautions to minimize the side effects of the medication. Successful performance of activities of daily living depends on competency in several areas including cognitive ability to sequence the steps of a task, physical ability to perform the task, perceptual ability to see what is done, and the executive ability to initiate and follow through with the task. Therefore, a problem in performance needs to be assessed and treated in a multidimensional manner.

Work with the psychologist and therapists to evaluate the patient's strengths and weaknesses. Implement and maintain a well-coordinated functional activities program that addresses these strengths and weaknesses.

Assist the family and/or caregivers in learning how to work with the patient to maintain his/her optimum level of function.

Cognitive Management

There is a great variability in the cognitive deficits evident in each person with TBI due to the diffuse nature of most injuries. Because of this variability, the cognitive management approaches also vary accordingly. A thorough neuropsychological evaluation as well as comprehensive systematic interdisciplinary evaluation are required to enable team members to develop the appropriate individualized program.

General treatment goals for cognitive management include: To challenge and channel spontaneous recovery; to maximize residual function; to compensate for loss; and to help the patient learn how to consciously process stimuli in an orderly, sequential manner; to evaluate the output; and to determine if change is necessary. Skills should be facilitated in a hierarchical order from the most basic first: Attention, selective attention, immediate memory, recent memory, sequential thought organization, reasoning, problem solving, and judgment. Unstructured, multiple modality treatment approaches may further exacerbate a patient's disorganized thinking. Controlling the rate, amount, duration, and complexity of stimulus input is critical to elicit structured and appropriate cognitive processing.

For decreased responsiveness develop a structured program of sensory stimulation. Work with one type of sensory stimulus at a time and eliminate extraneous stimuli. Use multisensory stimuli such as pictures, brightly colored objects, voice and music tapes, bells, clapping, different textures, tastes and scents, and position changes. Allow enough time for responses. Provide brief therapeutic sessions spaced throughout the day to avoid fatigue and overstimulation. Maintain consistent one-to-one interactions and interdisciplinary coordination. Provide simple, concrete, repetitive instructions.

For impaired memory and confusion provide structure, consistency, and repetition. Use orientation methods such as charts, clock, and daily log, and re-orient throughout the day. Emphasize old, over-learned, familiar skills. Maintain a safe, quiet environment. Use multiple modalities for teaching (auditory, visual, tactile) but keep approach structured and consistent. Pair old, familiar information with the new. Use memory aids and techniques such as notebooks and charts, watches, clocks, and calendars, categorization and pairing, and imagery. Place daily activities in exact, predictable sequence.

For impaired reasoning, abstract thinking, concept formation, and problem solving abilities present activities such as describing likenesses and differences, and analyzing potentially dangerous situations. Encourage the patient to participate in decision-making processes. Present activities such as categorizing tasks for color, size, and shape and organizing routine events by listing steps in process.

For impaired ability to generalize associate new learning with old and train in a situational environment. Start with simple tasks to assure success, then build complexity. Provide structured learning with frequent verbal cuing and demonstrations and then gradually decrease structure.

For executive function deficits assist the patient in developing short-term achievable goals, participating in the planning process, and following through with each step of the plan. Assist the patient in evaluating his/her progress and in making the necessary modifications in the plan.

For impaired insight and judgment provide the patient with information regarding the concept of brain damage and how it has affected him/her physically, cognitively, and emotionally. Encourage him/her to participate in peer group programs for sharing feelings, identifying problems, and working out solutions through group feedback.

For communication impairments work with the speech pathologist to implement and maintain an appropriate and consistent communication therapy program. Strategies include a combination of visual and auditory cuing for aphasia, oral motor strengthening and coordination exercises for dysarthria, breath support training to improve sustained voice volume, communication groups employing audio and video tapes and listener feedback for disorders of circumlocution and tangentiality, and communication devices to augment limited expressive skills.

Assist the family in understanding the patient's cognitive deficits. Assist them in learning how to effectively help him/her cope with the deficits and maximize his/her strengths.

Behavioral Management

Many types of behavioral disturbances may be manifested in the individual with TBI. The behavioral strategies selected will depend on the needs of the individual and his/her response to each. Cognitive problems such as impaired concentration and impaired receptive and expressive communication may indirectly contribute to behavior problems by exacerbating the individual's stress and frustration. Treatment measures include behavior modification,

psychotherapy, and psychoactive medications such as psychostimulants, tricyclic antidepressants, beta blockers, and lithium carbon-
ate. (Benzodiazepines and other sedatives can produce paradoxical
agitation. Psychostimulants may also lead to excessive stimulation
and agitation.) It is important when developing a treatment plan to
identify patterns of behavioral disturbance and the related exacerbating stimuli and to provide strategies for eliminating or modulat-
ing the patient's response. Also, strategies within the plan should
emphasize and provide positive reinforcement for appropriate behaviors rather than overly focusing on the maladaptive behaviors.

For agitation reduce the rate, duration, and complexity of stimuli. Provide a calm, nonthreatening, hazard-free environment. Avoid
restraints when possible. Allow the patient to talk out and walk out
restlessness. Project a calm attitude and eliminate non-verbal cues
that could be misinterpreted. Provide a structured, consistent activity plan and keep unexpected happenings to a minimum. Move the
patient gently into new activities—don't make sudden transitions.
When possible, eliminate or minimize potentially exacerbating
stimuli such as the physical discomfort of an indwelling catheter.

For impulsivity and reduced inhibition teach methods of self-control with a simple reward system. Provide immediate but non-punitive feedback on inappropriate behavior. Redirect the patient's attention to appropriate behavior. Provide a structured environment.
Discourage use of drugs.

For irritability and reduced tolerance to stress avoid excessive demands. Project calmness and consistency. Structure the environment so that unnecessary stress factors are removed. Assist the patient in learning relaxation techniques.

For emotional liability redirect the patient's attention to an unrelated area. Assist him/her in reducing the exacerbating factors of
stress and fatigue.

For obsessive behavior ignore it if possible. Confronting the individual may only lead to further obsession. Redirect his/her attention to a new idea or behavior. Praise his/her progress in applying
the new idea and/or behavior. Offer reassurance. Often obsessive behavior is a reflection of anxiety. Therefore, reducing the fear may
help relieve anxiety and enable the individual to move on to a different thought.

For delusional behavior state the facts in a calm, nondefensive
manner, but do not attempt to challenge the patient or argue with
irrationality. This type of behavior is a result of his/her inability to

pick up the appropriate cues and come to a logical conclusion. Therefore, attempts for a rational discussion of the issue are unlikely to succeed and may exacerbate the behavior.

For egocentrism and social inappropriateness provide group therapy experiences and ongoing feedback on the patient's impact on others. Avoid withdrawing from the individual and encourage consideration of others. Do not relinquish everything to his/her demands. Do not expect sensitivity and insight regarding your rights and feelings.

For depression, apathy, and withdrawal work with the psychologist and other disciplines to provide ongoing support and encouragement for the patient. Structure activities to facilitate his/her involvement. Provide individual and group opportunities for the individual to discuss feelings and frustrations. Administer psychostimulant or tricyclic antidepressant medication as ordered. Observe and record therapeutic effectiveness and side effects. Also, be aware that tricyclic antidepressants may affect the seizure threshold.

For sexuality concerns see pages 93–108.

Assist family members in understanding the TBI-related behavior changes experienced by the patient. Assist them in learning to effectively cope with these changes.

Perceptual Deficits Management

Somatagnosia, unilateral neglect, agnosia, apraxia, anosognosia, alterations in spatial and depth perception, and temporal disorders are some of the most frequently encountered perceptual deficits in persons with TBI. (Refer to pages 167–168 for further guidelines on managing perceptual deficits.)

Coordinate a therapy program with the occupational and physical therapists to remediate or compensate for the patient's perceptual deficits: Provide instruction in visual scanning methods to compensate for visual field deficits; use a full-length mirror to provide visual feedback for the individual with body schema disturbances; use verbal or written cues instead of gestures to assist the individual with visual-spatial problems. Teach functional skills in the associated setting using multiple teaching modalities. Employ compensatory strategies such as alternative positioning and assistive equipment to enhance abilities. Provide ongoing positive reinforcement for the patient's efforts. Maintain consistency in treatment procedures.

Assist the family in understanding the patient's perceptual deficits and the rationale for the recommended remedial and compensatory strategies.

Family Support

Family members often become isolated from friends and other outside contacts because of the patient's socially unacceptable behavior. They may suffer emotional and physical abuse due to the patient's lack of control, reduced tolerance to stress, and lack of empathy. They are often exhausted due to the constant physical and emotional demands of caring for the individual with TBI. In addition, old problems such as marital discord, parent-child friction, and poor communication may be intensified with the major lifestyle changes brought on by the injury. Differing expectations and conflicting methods of coping may further add to the feelings of stress, anger, guilt, fatigue, and depression experienced by family members.

Provide the family members with opportunities to ventilate their feelings in a safe, supportive environment. Provide information on the pathophysiology, manifestations, management, and recovery possibilities of TBI. Provide information for national and local community resource and support groups such as the National Head Injury Foundation, 333 Turnpike Road, Southborough, Massachusetts 01772. Refer family members for professional counseling when indicated.

FUTURE IMPLICATIONS

Recovery of function following brain damage is a very complex process. It consists of a number of mechanisms interacting in various combinations at different points in time. Understanding of the specific mechanisms of recovery is limited at present. Attempts to identify these mechanisms are further complicated by the difficulty in separating the effects of rehabilitation intervention strategies and the effects of the brain's intrinsic recovery process.

It is hoped that with ongoing research, progress will be made in understanding the specific mechanisms involved in brain damage and recovery and in identifying the processing specialties of individual brain systems and the processing requirements for performance of specific tasks. With this expanded knowledge base strategies such as functional substitution and pharmacological treatment may become more universally and effectively used within the rehabilitation setting.

REFERENCES

Baggerly, J. (1986). Rehabilitation of the adult with head trauma. *Nursing Clinics of North America, 21*:581–583.

Burke, W. (1988). Altered behavior analysis in head injury rehabilitation. *Rehabilitation Nursing, 13*(4):186–188.

Cooper, P. (1986). *Head injury.* Baltimore: Williams and Wilkins.

Deutsch, P., and Fralish, K. (1988). *Innovations in head injury rehabilitation.* New York: Matthew Bender.

Gibbs, J. (1987). Rehabilitation in head injury: A case study. *Rehabilitation Nursing 12*(3):137–138.

Herbel, K., Schermerhorn, L., and Howard, J. (1990). Management of agitated head injured patients: A survey of current techniques. *Rehabilitation Nursing, 15*(2):66–69.

Howard, M. (1988). Behavioral management in the acute care rehabilitation setting. *The Journal of Head Trauma Rehabilitation, 3*(3):14–22.

Hyunok, D., Sahagian, D., Schuster, L., and Sheridan, S. (1988). Head trauma rehabilitation: Program evaluation. *Rehabilitation Nursing, 13*(2): 71–75.

Kreutzer, J. (Ed.). (1989). Cognitive rehabilitation. *The Journal of Head Trauma Rehabilitation, 4*(3):1–84.

Long, D. (1989). Issues in behavioral neurology in brain injury. In D. Ellis and A. Christensen (Eds.). *Neuropsychological Treatment After Brain Injury.* Norwell, MA: Kluwer Academic Publishers.

Manifold, S. (1986). Craniocerebral trauma: A review of primary and secondary injury and therapeutic modalities. *Focus on Critical Care, 13*(2):22–35.

Meier, M., Benton, A., and Diller, L. (1987). *Neuropsychological rehabilitation.* New York: Guilford Press.

Patterson, T., and Sargent, M. (1990). Behavioral management of the agitated head trauma client. *Rehabilitation Nursing, 15*(5):248–249.

Rosenthal, M., Griffith, E., Bond, M., and Miller, J. (1990). *Rehabilitation of the adult and child with traumatic brain injury* (2nd ed.). Philadelphia: F. A. Davis Company.

Sherman, D. (1990). Managing acute head injury. *Nursing 90, 20*(4):46–51.

Simon, R., and Sayre, J. (1987). *Strategies in head injury management.* Norwalk, CT: Appleton and Lange.

Sohlberg, M., and Mateer, C. (1989). *Introduction to cognitive rehabilitation: Theory and practice.* New York: Guilford Press.

Szekeres, S., Szekeres, Y., and Cohen, S. (1987). A framework for cognitive rehabilitation therapy. In M. Ylwasker and E. Gobble (Eds.). *Community reentry for head injured adults.* Boston: College Hill Press.

Uomoto, J. (1990). Neuropsychological Assessment and training. In F. Kottke and F. Lehmann (Eds.). *Handbook of physical medicine and rehabilitation.* (4th Ed). Philadelphia: W. B. Saunders Co.

Vogenthaler, D. (1987). Overview of head injury: Its consequences in rehabilitation. *Brain Injury, 11*(1):113–127.

Spinal Cord Injury Management

9

OBJECTIVES

After completing this chapter, the reader will be able to:

- Compare and contrast the types of spinal cord injuries (SCI) and related impairments.
- Describe the autonomic changes associated with SCI and discuss related nursing interventions.
- Describe the respiratory, cardiovascular, urological, gastrointestinal, and integumentary complications associated with SCI and describe preventive and treatment measures.
- Discuss interventions for maximizing the patient's functional potential and for preventing musculoskeletal complications.
- Discuss interventions to enhance the patient's coping skills and facilitate psychosocial adjustment.

INTRODUCTION

Spinal cord injury (SCI) is a catastrophic event with far reaching consequences for the victim, family and friends, and for society as a whole. According to the National SCI Statistical Center there are between 7000 and 10,000 new cases of traumatic SCI each year in the United States, with an estimated prevalence of 200,000. Over half of this population is between the ages of 15 and 30, and 80 percent are males. The most common causes of traumatic SCI, in decreasing order of incidence, are vehicular accidents, falls, gunshot wounds, and diving accidents. Individuals who sustain SCIs need the expertise and the support of rehabilitation nurses working with other rehabilitation team members to assist in maximizing functional abilities, preventing complications, and facilitating psychosocial adjustment.

PATHOPHYSIOLOGY

Vertebral Injuries

The degree and type of force exerted on the spine at the time of an accident are determining factors as to whether a vertebral injury occurs. Sudden hyperflexion and rotation, as seen in many vehicular accidents, frequently results in a fracture dislocation. C5-6 and T12-L1 are the most common sites for fracture dislocation. Such a fracture is unstable due to posterior longitudinal ligament damage, and usually causes the greatest degree of cord damage.

High-impact longitudinal trauma, as seen after a long-distance fall, often results in a compression fracture. This is a more stable fracture as the posterior ligament and posterior bony elements remain intact. The most common sites for a compression fracture are also C5-6 and T12-L1.

A hyperextension injury from a fall or vehicular accident is found most often in the older person with a narrowed spinal canal due to osteoarthritis in the spine. C4-5 is the most common injury site. Skeletal damage is seen in the anterior ligament rather than in the vertebral column. If spinal cord damage occurs, it is primarily in the center of the cord. Though varying degrees of spinal cord damage usually accompany vertebral fractures and dislocations, not all SCIs are associated with vertebral injuries. The cord may also be damaged by a bullet or a knife wound.

Effects of Injury on Spinal Cord and Related Research

The spinal cord is rarely physically transected by any of these injuries. The damage results from an autodestruction process that begins at the time of the initial insult. At the time, petechial hemorrhages occur in the gray matter. Within 1 to 2 hours, extravasation of fluid, red blood cells, and lymphocytes extend through the gray matter. The hemorrhages, edema, and metabolic products acting together result in ischemia and necrosis of the spinal neurons. In response to the trauma the body increases the production of norepinephrine and endorphins. These, in turn, cause vascular changes which result in further hypoxia and necrosis. Within 4 hours after injury 40 percent of the gray matter and adjacent white matter at the injury site may be necrosed. Within 24 hours the continuation of the destructive process results in extensive necrotic changes. Edema secondary to the inflammatory process compresses the cord and further increases the ischemic damage. While there is usually a stabilization of the destructive processes within 48 hours, progressive edema can extend the damage up to 72 hours.

Many research projects are being conducted currently in an attempt to isolate these destructive factors and develop treatments to counteract their effects. The following experimental methods are being used at various medical centers in the United States: Alpha methytyrosine (AMT), reserpine, or levodopa administered within 15 minutes of injury to counteract the effects of norepinephrine; naloxone or thyrotropin releasing hormone (TRH) administered within the first hour of injury to counteract the effects of the catecholamines and endorphins. Further work is needed before conclusions can be made on their long-term benefits.*

Other modalities under investigation include peripheral nerve grafts to enhance the regrowth environment, administration of nerve growth factor and thyroid hormones to increase anabolic actions, fetal tissue transplants to replace neurons, and electrical stimulation to enhance neuron growth. There is no conclusive evidence in support of any of these modalities at the present time.

Spinal Shock

Immediately following SCI there is diminished excitability of the isolated cord characterized by loss of vasomotor and reflex activity below the level of injury. This state is referred to as spinal or neuro-

---

*On March 30, 1990, the National Institute of Health released the results of a several year multicenter study of the use of methylprednisolone. When given within 8 hours of injury, high intravenous doses of this drug (given over a period of 24 hours) can reduce the motor and sensory losses associated with SCI. It is thought to act by stabilizing nerve cell membranes and protecting them from further injury after the initial trauma.

genic shock. The transient depression of reflex activity is due to the sudden withdrawal of facilitating influences from the supraspinal centers. With the disruption of transmission between the higher centers and the synapses of the cord, conduction is impossible. Spinal shock usually lasts from 3 days to several weeks. The return of reflex activity in individuals with UMN lesions signals the end of spinal shock. If the injury is below the conus medularris (LMN lesion) there is no evidence of reflex activity and the skeletal and visceral muscles remain flaccid permanently.

After spinal shock has resolved, the extent of further neurological recovery is variable. With minimal neurological damage recovery may be nearly complete within a few days. With a moderate degree of neurological damage, recovery may take place over a period of 12 to 36 months. With extensive neurological damage, no significant recovery can be expected.

Injury Classifications

Complete-Incomplete Classification

Neurological manifestations depend on the location and severity of the injury. In a complete SCI there is total sensory and motor function loss resulting from a complete interruption of the ascending and descending tracts below the level of the lesion. With an incomplete injury there is preservation of some of the sensory and/or motor function depending on the specific tracts that are damaged and spared. Incomplete injuries are categorized according to the area of damage: Central, lateral, anterior, or peripheral (Figure 9-1).

A central cord injury results when there is more cellular destruction in the center of the cord than in the periphery. There is greater paralysis and sensory loss in the upper extremities than in the lower extremities, as these upper extremity functions are mediated by the medial corticospinal tracts in the cord. The mechanism of injury is hyperextension, usually with no vertebral damage. The syndrome is seen most often in older people who have loss of ligament elasticity and cervical canal narrowing from arthritic changes.

A Brown-Sequard syndrome results form an anterior-posterior hemisection of the cord, as in a stabbing or gunshot injury. Below the level of injury there is a loss of motor function, proprioception, deep touch, and vibration on the ipsilateral side and loss of pain, temperature, pressure, and light touch on the contralateral side due

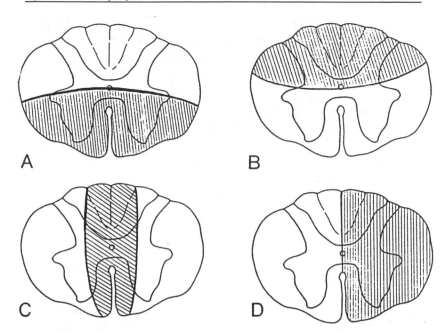

FIGURE 9-1 A: Anterior cord syndrome; B: Posterior cord syndrome; C: Central cord syndrome; D: Brown-Sequard syndrome. (Buchanan, L., and Nawoczenski, D. *Spinal Cord Injury: Concepts and Management Approaches*. Baltimore: Williams and Wilkins, 1987.)

to the crossing over of the descending motor tracts at the medulla and the ascending sensory tracts crossing over at the dorsal root level.

An anterior cord syndrome results from a flexion injury that damages the anterior portions of the white and gray matter of the cord which affects the major corticospinal (motor) tracts and, to a lesser extent, some of the sensory tracts. There is paralysis and loss of pain, temperature, and deep pressure with preservation of proprioception and light touch. In a posterior cord syndrome there is a loss of the sensory modalities of proprioception, discrimination, and vibration while the motor tracts in the anterior cord may be largely unaffected.

Cauda equina injuries involve peripheral nerves rather than the spinal cord directly. Since peripheral nerves possess a regenerating capacity that the cord does not, there is a better prognosis for recovery in these injuries. Patterns of sensory and motor deficits are highly variable and asymmetric in cauda equina injuries.

Motor Neuron and Disability Classification

Injuries may be classified as upper motor neuron (UMN) or lower motor neuron (LMN). An UMN lesion occurs above T12/L1 and disrupts motor axons in the corticospinal tracts resulting in paralysis and increased muscle tone below the level of injury and intact reflexes which are not influenced by supraspinal control. A LMN lesion occurs at or below L1 or in a central or longitudinal cord injury resulting in a flaccid paralysis below the level of injury, disrupted reflex arcs, and absent reflexes. A mixed injury occurs at T12/L1 with manifestations such as flaccid bladder and spastic sphincter or spastic lower extremities and flaccid bladder.

Neurological Classification

In 1983 the American Spinal Injury Association (ASIA) developed standards for neurological classification of SCI patients in an attempt to provide a more consistent method of communication. These standards are based on the premise that the level of injury is the lowest level in which functional motor power (the ability to accomplish full range of motion against gravity but without resistance) and sensation remain intact after SCI (Table 9-1).

Systemic Effects and Related Complications

Autonomic Hyperreflexia (Dysreflexia)

Autonomic hyperreflexia is a life threatening complication encountered in individuals with spinal cord lesions above T6. It is the result of increased autonomic activity caused by a noxious stimulus below the level of injury. This stimulus is most often a distended bladder or bowel. Urinary stones, severe bladder infections, decubitus ulcers, and ingrown toenails are some of the other stimulants that may initiate the autonomic response.

Impulses travel from the site of the stimulus up the spinothalamic and posterior columns until they are blocked at the level of the lesion. Here a sympathetic reflex is activated and results in massive reflex sympathetic nerve overactivity below the level of the lesion. There is arteriolar spasm in the skin and viscera increasing peripheral resistance. The individual experiences a severe headache as

TABLE 9-1 Frankel Scale—Functional Classification

A. COMPLETE
  No preservation of motor or sensory function.
B. INCOMPLETE—PRESERVED SENSATION ONLY
  Preservation of any demonstrable sensation below the level of injury,
  except phantom sensations.
C. INCOMPLETE—PRESERVED MOTOR NONFUNCTIONAL
  Preserved motor function without useful purpose (grade 1 or 2);
  sensory function may or may not be preserved.
D. INCOMPLETE—PRESERVED MOTOR FUNCTIONAL
  Preserved voluntary motor function that is functionally useful
  (grade 3 or better).
E. COMPLETE RECOVERY
  Complete return of all motor and sensory function, but may still have
  abnormal reflexes.

From "Standards for Neurological Classification of Spinal Injury Patients," American Spinal Injury Association, November 1983.

his/her blood pressure rapidly rises. The hypertension stimulates pressure receptors in the aortic and carotid sinus. The vasomotor center in the medulla then sends parasympathetic impulses via the vagus nerve in an attempt to lower the blood pressure. The resulting vasodilatation causes the individual to become flushed, sweat profusely above the lesion level, and develop nasal congestion. The vagus stimulation also causes cardiac slowing.

Because the impulses from the vasomotor center that would cause splanchnic pooling and allow a decrease in blood pressure are blocked at the level of the lesion, their effects are only manifested above this level. Consequently, the sympathetic vasoconstrictive response continues to elevate the blood pressure until the precipitating stimulus is removed. Without rapid intervention the greatly elevated pressure can result in a seizure and/or an intracranial or subarachnoid hemorrhage or fatal cardiac arrhythmias.

The following is a review of other systemic effects and complications of SCI. The etiologies are in parentheses.

1. *Cardiovascular:* Bradycardia (unopposed vagal stimulation); reduced cardiac output (bradycardia); hypotension (loss of vasoconstrictive tone and decreased cardiac output); cardiac arrest and arrhythmias (unopposed vagal stimulation, hypoxia, and electrolyte imbalance); deep venous thrombosis and pul-

monary embolism (decreased vascular and muscle tone, increased coagulability, immobility, vascular injury).

2. *Thermoregulation:* Poikilothermia (disruption between hypothalamus, ANS, and cardiovascular system).

3. *Respiratory:* Respiratory arrest—primarily in cervical injuries (respiratory muscle fatigue/paralysis and/or phrenic nerve damage, associated chest injuries, respiratory infections, abdominal distention, pre-existing respiratory conditions); atelectasis, pneumonia, and acute bronchial obstruction (inability to move secretions as a result of partial or complete paralysis of respiratory muscles and from immobility).

4. *Urological:* Renal ischemia during spinal shock phase (decreased cardiac output and hypotension); diuresis during first days post injury (neurohormonal and electrolyte disruptions); bladder dysfunction (neurological damage); infection, calculi, reflux, and hydronephrosis (see pages 51–68).

5. *Gastrointestinal:* Paralytic ileus during first days post injury (ANS disruption); ulcers and GI bleeding during first days post injury (stress response, steroid administration, and excess hydrochloric acid production).

6. *Horners Syndrome* (paralysis of cervical portion of sympathetic chain).

7. *Sensory changes and pain:* Loss of sensation and/or abnormal sensations (interruption of ascending sensory tracts); somatic pain (medical condition or irritation of nerve roots); central pain with undetermined etiology.

8. *Integumentary:* Altered skin integrity (sensory loss; immobility; temperature and sweating irregularities; cardiovascular dysfunction with vasodilation, tissue hypoxia, and edema; bowel and bladder dysfunctions with incontinence; nutritional inadequacies with anemia, hypoalbuminemia, and negative nitrogen balance; medical complications with decreased resistance and increased susceptibility to infection; musculoskeletal complications such as spasticity and contractures; medications that cause immunosuppression or coagulation abnormalities; psychosocial issues such as depression, lack of family support, financial constraints, and substance abuse).

9. *Musculoskeletal:* Paralysis/paresis (interruption of descending motor tracts); spasticity (UMN reflex activity with exacerbating factors such as pain, pressure sores, manipulation of muscle belly, ingrown toenails); heterotopic ossification and patho-

logical fracture (bone absorption from lack of weight-bearing activities).

NURSING INTERVENTIONS

Assessment

Health History

- Mechanism of injury, time since injury, and associated injuries.
- Systems review indicating problems experienced since injury.
- Pre-existing conditions or diseases such as ankylosing spondylitis or osteoarthritis of the spine.
- Current medications.
- Known allergies.
- Personal history including diet, sleep, smoking, and exercise patterns and psychosocial status.

Physical Assessment Findings

- Partial or complete loss of motor function below level of injury (See Table 9-2).
- Loss of reflex activity below level of injury in spinal shock stage.
- Partial or complete loss of pain, temperature, touch, vibration, and proprioception below level of injury.
- Atonic bladder in spinal shock stage, reflex or autonomous presentation in later stages.
- Paralytic ileus in spinal shock stage, reflex or autonomous presentation in later stages.
- Hypotension and bradycardia (most pronounced in injuries above T5-T6).
- Absence of independent respiratory function (injuries above C4).
- Impaired deep breathing and decreased or absent chest expansion ability with decreased vital capacity and tidal volume (cervical and upper thoracic injuries).
- Impaired coughing ability and decreased or absent abdominal movement.
- Impaired sweating response.

TABLE 9-2 Spinal Cord Segments and Corresponding Muscles/Movement

Spinal Cord Segment	Muscle(s)	Movement
C1-3	neck muscles	limited head control
C4	diaphragm	diaphragmatic breathing
	trapezius	shoulder shrug
C5	deltoid	shoulder abduction
	partial biceps	partial elbow flexion
C6	extensor carpi radialis	wrist extension
	biceps	elbow flexion
C7	triceps	elbow extension
	extensor digitorum	finger extension
C8	flexor digitorum	finger flexion
T1	hand intrinsics	finger abduction, adduction
T2-T12	intercostals	deeper inhalation
T6-T12	abdominals	forceful exhalation
		increased trunk stability
L1-L2	iliopsoas	hip flexion
L2-L3	hip adductors	hip adduction
L3-L4	quadriceps femoris	knee extension
L4-L5	tibialis anterior	ankle extension
L5	extensor hallucis longus	great toe extension
S1	gastrocnemius/soleus	plantar flexion
	hamstrings	knee flexion
S1-S2	flexor digitorum	toe flexion
S2-S4	bladder, lower bowel	elimination

- Evidence of decreased level of consciousness, cranial nerve dysfunction, elevated intracranial pressure (in presence of concurrent head injury).

*Diagnostic Tests**

- Spinal x-rays and tomograms to visualize vertebral fracture or dislocation
- Myelogram and computed tomography (CT scan) to visualize presence of pressure on spinal cord.
- Epidurogram to visualize any lacerated tissue fragments that may have been propelled into spinal canal.

---

*It is essential that the vertebral column in the newly injured person be kept immobilized in proper alignment throughout all diagnostic procedures.

- Somatosensory evoked potential (SEPs) and motor evoked potentials (MEPs) to determine if there is any electrical continuity between the peripheral nerves, spinal cord, and brain.

Nursing Diagnoses: Actual or Potential

1. Impaired physical mobility related to paresis, plegia, spasticity.
2. Altered comfort: Pain related to altered sensory responses.
3. Sensory alterations: Kinesthetic, tactile related to altered sensory reception and transmission.
4. Potential for injury related to sensory and motor deficits.
5. Self-care deficit related to sensory and motor deficits, pain.
6. Activity intolerance related to deconditioning and/or motor deficits, pain.
7. Altered cardiovascular responses: Hypotension, dependent edema, and bradycardia related to ANS disruption and positioning.
8. Altered tissue perfusion: Peripheral related to impaired venous circulation to extremities.
9. Respiratory dysfunction: Hypoventilation related to respiratory muscle paralysis; pulmonary congestion and atelectasis related to muscle paralysis and immobility.
10. Impaired skin integrity related to immobility, mechanical factors, altered nutritional status, impaired sensation, impaired circulation.
11. Altered bowel elimination: Incontinence, constipation related to neurological dysfunction, immobility, lack of privacy, inadequate diet, medication side effects.
12. Altered nutritional status: Less than body requirements related to anorexia, inability to feed self.
13. Altered urinary elimination: Incontinence, retention related to neurological dysfunction.
14. Dysreflexia related to bladder distention, calculi, infection; bowel impaction; decubitus or other noxious stimuli.
15. Sexual dysfunction related to biopsychosocial alteration of sexuality, absence of role models, lack of privacy, lack of knowledge.
16. Social isolation related to sensory and motor deficits, self-concept disturbances, environmental barriers.

17. Disturbance in self-concept: Body image, self-esteem.
18. Anxiety related to threat to self-concept, role functioning, and interaction patterns; unmet needs.
19. Grieving: Dysfunctional or anticipatory related to actual or perceived losses.
20. Ineffective individual coping related to inadequate information, inadequate support, multiple life changes.
21. Knowledge deficit related to SCI management.

Expected Outcomes: Patient and/or Family

1. The individual maintains functional alignment and sustains no complications of immobility.
2. The individual uses correct techniques to facilitate mobility and to compensate for motor and sensory deficits.
3. The individual is comfortable as evidenced by verbal statements and/or body language.
4. The individual is free of injury.
5. The individual reestablishes role functions and socialization patterns and engages in self-care activities consistent with sensory and motor limitations.
6. The individual employs compensatory measures to maintain cardiovascular stability.
7. The individual remains free of vascular complications.
8. The individual's lungs remain clear.
9. The individual's skin integrity is restored or maintained.
10. The individual's bowel and bladder patterns are stabilized.
11. The individual is free of urinary and bowel complications.
12. The individual is free of dysreflexia.
13. The individual maintains nutritional status as evidenced by stable body weight and normal hematocrit, hemoglobin, and serum protein.
14. The individual verbalizes perception of himself/herself as a sexual being.
15. The individual experiences decreased anxiety and improved self-concept as evidenced by verbal statements and/or body language.
16. The individual verbalizes and demonstrates an understanding of SCI management.

Planning and Implementation

(Include the family, significant other, and/or caregiver in the teaching interventions.)

Neurological Management

During acute and early rehabilitation stages, surgical intervention may be necessary if there is cord compression by bony fragments or severe dislocation. External stabilizing devices may be used following spinal surgery or in place of surgery. For cervical injuries, skeletal traction may be used with Crutchfield, Cone Vinke, or Gardner Wells tongs. Other devices used to maintain cervical stabilization include a sterno-occipital mandibular immobilizer (SOMI or Guilford brace), two-piece molded plastic collars or jackets with neck support, and halo traction. For thoracolumbar stabilization, molded plastic jackets, Jewett braces, or Knight Taylor corsets may be used.

Prepare the patient physically and psychologically for surgical procedure and/or application of stabilizing device. Provide post-op care as ordered. Provide preventive skin care including tong or pin site care when applicable. Maintain positioning appropriate for patient's vertebral stability, respiratory, and integumentary status.

Assist the patient in learning about the pathophysiology, manifestations, and therapeutic management of SCI.

Cardiovascular Management

During acute and early rehabilitation stages, minimize the risk of cardiac arrhythmias by maintaining fluid and electrolyte balance and adequate oxygenation, by alleviating pain, and by treating anxiety.

Prevent excess vagal stimulation and sinus arrest by limiting respiratory suctioning to a maximum of 15 seconds with pre- and post-oxygen administration. Avoid turning the patient rapidly. Administer medication as ordered (usually atropine or isoproterenol [Isuprel]). Observe and record the patient's response. Take precautions to minimize the side effects of the medication.

Implement and maintain DVT and PE prevention measures: frequent turns, proper positioning, lower extremity range of motion exercises and heel cord stretching, deep breathing exercises, thigh-length elastic stocking, and prophylactic anticoagulants as

prescribed. Observe for signs and symptoms of increased calf and/
or thigh measurements, low grade fever, increased spasticity, local-
ized discomfort, vital sign changes and respiratory distress. Observe
and record patient's response to the medication. Take precautions
to minimize side effects of the medication.

Implement measures to manage orthostatic hypotension, including use of abdominal binder and thigh-length elastic stockings and
slow elevation from a reclining position. Severe hypotension problems may require fluid supplementation and an order for ephedrine
sulfate with sodium chloride.

Minimize dependent edema with elastic stockings and lower extremity elevation.

Assist the patient in learning orthostatic hypotension, DVT, and
dependent edema preventive measures and in proper suctioning
technique when applicable.

Respiratory Management

Implement measures to prevent hypoventilation, hypoxia, and
respiratory arrest including assistive coughing, intermittent positive pressure breathing, incentive spirometer or blow bottles, a high
fluid intake, humidified environment, and frequent position
changes. (Note: The prone position can decrease tidal volume and vital capacity and block inspiration. When sidelying, the person with
a hemidiaphragm should be positioned with the weak side upper-
most to maximize the diaphragmatic recoil. With abdominal muscle
paralysis [cervical and high thoracic injuries] a person's vital capacity decreases 30 percent with sitting 60 degrees or higher. An abdominal binder facilitates diaphragmatic excursion by limiting the
pull of the abdominal viscera.)

To enable the ventilator-dependent quadriplegic to spend some
time off the ventilator, coordinate a program with the chest therapist that will assist the patient in strengthening the sternocleido-
mastoid and scalenus muscles and in learning independent head
support and glossopharyngeal breathing (using the mouth and
throat to force air into the lungs). A pneumobelt is effective for
some people with partial diaphragm function. It works with
negative pressure that produces a forceful exhalation and a passive
inhalation.

Assist the patient in learning respiratory management measures
including assisted cough, positioning, chest therapy, signs and

symptoms of complications, tracheostomy care, equipment care and suctioning if applicable.

For a person with a C1 or C2 injury and intact phrenic nerve the diaphragmatic (phrenic nerve) pacer provides an alternative to the ventilator. The pacer has an external battery operated unit and antennae which activate internal implants, stimulating the phrenic nerve and subsequently the diaphragm. To be a candidate for a phrenic pacemaker an individual must have LMN preservation so that the reflex arc is able to react to the electric charge of the pacemaker. Potential candidates must undergo fluoroscopy and transcutaneous nerve conduction studies to determine phrenic nerve response to stimulation and to visualize diaphragmatic excursion. Potential complications from the implant include wire displacement, equipment failure, and site infection.

Prepare the patient for diagnostic tests and for the implant procedure. Assist the patient, family, and other care providers in learning equipment operation, patient positioning;, signs and symptoms of respiratory failure and site infection, battery maintenance and charging, and use of the rebreathing bag.

Urological Management

Implement measures to prevent urological complications. Assist the patient in learning preventive and treatment measures. (See pages 51–68.)

Gastrointestinal Management

During the acute/early rehabilitation stage, implement measures to determine the presence and resolution of an ileus and to prevent ileus-related complications: Abdominal girth measurements, bowel sound monitoring, nasogastric tube placement with low pressure suctioning, nasogastric tube placement with low pressure suctioning, and an alternate method of nutrition and hydration until GI motility returns.

After the resolution of the ileus, implement a bowel management program to prevent incontinence and constipation. Assist the patient in learning preventive and treatment measures. (See pages 69–80.)

Provide early detection of GI bleeding with ongoing assessment of vital signs, stool guaics, gastric aspirations, and hemoglobin and hematocrit. Implement measures to decrease the incidence of ulcers and GI bleeding by administering antacids and histamine H2 antagonists (usually ranitidine/Zantac or cimetidine/Tagamet) as ordered. Observe and record the patient's response. Take precautions to minimize the side effects of the medication.

Autonomic Hyperreflexia Management

Elevate the head of the bed if the patient is in a recumbent position.

Check for and eliminate the precipitating noxious stimulus when possible. The most likely stimuli are a distended or irritated bladder, a distended bowel, or a skin lesion below the level of injury. If patency cannot be restored to an indwelling catheter with a 30cc. irrigation, replace the catheter. If a stool disimpaction is required use a local anesthetic cream or jelly in the rectum prior to the disimpaction procedure. if a skin lesion is present apply a topical anesthetic to the site to reduce the stimulation.

Administer medications as ordered if the noxious stimulus cannot be removed or if the symptoms persist after the cause has been removed. Hydralazine (Apresoline), phenoxybenzamine (Dibenzyline), nifedipine (Procardia) or phentolamine (Regitine) may be used. Monitor and record the patient's response.

After hyperreflexia has been resolved, continue to monitor vital signs every 4 hours for 24 hours to detect rebound hypertension.

Assist the patient in learning the signs and symptoms, causes, treatment, and prevention of hyperreflexia.

Integumentary Management

Identify and minimize risk factors with pressure relief and shearing prevention measures, nutritional supplementation as needed, optimum hygiene, proper clothing, and treatment of health and psychological problems.

When a skin breakdown is present, implement a wound care program based on the grade, location, and general status of the sore (Table 9-3).

Assist the patient in learning pressure relief measures, proper positioning techniques, how to perform a skin check, how to care for a decubitus, and how to employ other preventive measures through diet, skin care, clothing selection, and safety precautions.

TABLE 9-3 Pressure Sore Management

Grade*	Treatment	Advantages/Disadvantages
I	1. Normal saline or neutral cleanser.	1. Soap and alcohol are too drying and alkaline residue from soap disrupts skin's protective acid mantle.
	2. a. Skin barrier if skin intact b. Moisture vapor permeable transparent (MVPT) dressing for open wound.	2. a. Protects skin. b. Protects open sore from bacteria and from premature drying.
II	1. Cleanse is in Grade I. If wound infected use antiseptic solution.	1. a. Povidone iodine has antibacterial properties and acts as wound irritant to stimulate granulation tissue. It is very drying, can irritate health tissue, and cause systemic toxicity. b. Hydrogen peroxide (H_2O_2), acetic acid, and Dakin's solution have minimal healing effect, may harm fragile granulation tissue, and increase wound bleeding.
	2. a. MVPT dressing.	2. a. Protects open sore from bacteria and premature drying.
	b. Moist saline dressing.	b. Promotes epithelization in wound bed.
	c. Hydrocolloid and hydrophilic absorption dressings for draining wound.	c. Have antiinfective properties, stimulate growth of granulation tissue, and absorb exudate.
III and IV	1. For non-necrotic wound cleanse and dress as in Grade II (eliminate MVPT dressing).	1. As above #1 and 2.
	2. a. For necrotic wound cleanse as in Grade II.	2. a. As above #1.
	b. Assist with surgical debridement.	b. Necrotic tissue and eschars decrease effectiveness of treatment measures.

(Continued)

TABLE 9-3 *(Continued)*

Grade*	Treatment	Advantages/Disadvantages
	c. Enzyme preparation.	c. Provides enzymatic debriding action—use antibacterial powder with enzyme preparation as bacteria proliferate when necrotic tissue liquifies.
	d. Wet to dry dressing with wide mesh gauze.	d. Provides mechanical debriding action.
	3. Assist with preparatory measures for surgical repair.	
	a. Nutritional supplementation and blood transfusions.	a. To facilitate recovery action.
	b. Spasticity management measures.	b. To avoid damaging surgical site.
	c. Systemic antibiotic administration.	c. To eliminate wound and systemic infection.

*Grade I—epidermis to dermal junction; II—epidermal and dermal layers and adipose tissue; III—through adipose tissue and muscle; IV—destruction through soft tissue to or onto bone.

Musculoskeletal Management

Table 9-4 describes some of the skills possible for different functional levels of complete SCI. These descriptions are presented only as general guidelines; there are many psychological and physical factors that will influence each person's functional capabilities.

Functional electrical stimulation (FES) is one of the latest developments in musculoskeletal management. It consists of electrical stimulation to certain muscles with a biofeedback component. The process is controlled by computers. The purpose of FES is to improve muscle strength and/or to prevent atrophy, to improve functional abilities, to control spasticity, and to increase cardiovascular endurance. Ambulation is the most publicized area of FES success. However, this is only available at selected research centers at this time. Other FES equipment is becoming more available in regional SCI centers and for home use in the forms of the Regys and Ergys ergometers. Ergometers are computerized bikes that send a sequence of electric currents to paralyzed muscles in the lower extremities. This stimulates them to move the bike pedals against re-

TABLE 9-4 Neurological Levels and Functional Potential

Level	Activity
C1-4	Dependent in feeding, grooming, dressing, bathing, bowel and bladder routines, bed mobility, transfers, and transportation. Independent wheelchair propulsion with pneumatic or chin control and with electronically adapted communication and environmental control devices.
C1-3	Dependent on ventilation support.
C5	Independent feeding and grooming with adapted equipment. Dependent in dressing, bathing, bowel and bladder routines, and transportation. Requires assistance for bed mobility and transfers. Independent wheelchair propulsion in motorized chair and with electronically adapted communication and environmental control devices.
C6	Independent feeding, grooming, upper extremity dressing, bathing, bowel routine, and bed mobility—all with adapted equipment. Requires assistance for lower extremity dressing and bladder routine. Potentially independent transfers with transfer board. Independent manual wheelchair propulsion with plastic rims or lugs indoors. Independent driving with adapted van. Independent phone operation and page turning with equipment.
C7	Independent feeding, grooming and bathing with equipment. Potentially independent in upper and lower extremity dressing and bowel and bladder routines. Independent bed mobility, transfers with or without board, manual wheelchair propulsion, driving with adapted car or van and in communication activities.
C8-T1	Independent in all personal care activities, bed mobility, transfers, wheelchair propulsion, driving with adapted car or van, and in communication activities.
T2-T10	Independent in all activities. Ambulation with long leg braces and crutches or walker for exercise only (nonfunctional).
T11-L2	Independent in all activities. Potentially independent functional ambulation indoors with long leg braces and crutches.
L2-S3	Independent in all activities. Independent ambulation indoors and outdoors with short leg braces and crutches or canes.

sistance. Individuals with incomplete injuries and with injuries below T10 are not eligible candidates for the ergometer.

Coordinate and maintain an activities of daily living program with occupational and physical therapists to maximize the patient's functional abilities.

Provide resource and referral information to those individuals interested in FES (Corbet, 1985, pp. 15–16).

Coordinate a program of weight bearing and gentle range of motion exercises with the therapists to prevent/minimize heterotopic ossification. Administer medication as prescribed to control calcium deposition (diaphosphonate/Didronel). Observe and record the patient's response. Take precautions to minimize side effects of the medication.

Implement measures to prevent spasticity-exacerbating conditions such as pressure sores and urinary tract infections. Administer antispasticity medications as prescribed such as baclophen (Lioresal), diazepam (Valium), and dantrolene sodium (Dantrium). Observe and record the patient's response. Take precautions to minimize side effects of the medication. Work with physicians and therapists on a plan to minimize spasticity and prevent contractures using optimum positioning techniques, inhibiting techniques, and ROM exercises. Table 9-5 reviews spasticity management techniques.

TABLE 9-5 Spasticity Management Techniques

1. Proprioceptive neuromuscular facilitation: Breaks up abnormal patterns by using neurodevelopmental measures and stronger movements to overcome weaker movements.
2. Reflex inhibiting patterns: Abolishes abnormal patterns and reinforces correct movements.
3. Splinting: Inhibits abnormal patterns.
4. Icing: Facilitates override of spasticity.
5. Heat: Relaxes spastic muscles.
6. Balance activities: Help with righting and equilibrium reactions.
7. Pharmacologic agents: Lioresal acts on reflex pathways in spinal cord; Valium acts at brain, spinal cord, and muscle levels; Dantrium acts on skeletal muscles.
8. Motor point blocks: Block gamma motor fibers, making muscle spindles less sensitive to stretch but not affecting larger fibers.
9. Surgical procedures: Neurectomy, rhizotomy, tendon lengthening, dorsal column stimulator implantation.

Assist the patient in learning preventive positioning, range of motion exercises, medications (purpose, dosage, schedule, side effects, and precautions), and measures to prevent spasticity-exacerbating conditions, and the correct use of adaptive equipment.

Psychological Management

Be honest and realistic with the patient and family regarding the injury consequences and rehabilitative potentials.

Ascertain the meaning of the patient associates with the disability and loss of specific body functions. Provide opportunities for ventilation and sharing of feelings and experiences. Assist the patient in understanding the effects of past experiences and responses to the current situation.

Allow the patient to mourn his/her losses by being a sensitive and supportive listener.

Assist the patient to regain self-confidence and a positive self-image by collaborating with him/her on realistic goal setting that capitalizes on personal strengths and resources. Provide education opportunities to increase the patient's understanding of his/her condition and to increase his/her sense of control. Promote self-esteem by providing positive feedback on learning and self-improvement efforts.

Provide a supportive environment with built-in flexibility to allow the patient to begin to explore without fear of failure.

Assist the patient in coping with the stress of rehabilitation and of the disability by providing consistent information, acknowledging progress, teaching relaxation techniques, and making counseling referrals when indicated.

Refer the patient and family to a resource group such as the National Spinal Cord Injury Association (600 West Cummings Park, Suite 200, Woburn, MA 01801) for further support and information.

Sexual Counseling

Assist the individual to maintain his/her sexual identity by minimizing the number of embarrassing, intrusive procedures and exposures; supporting the maintenance of physical appearance; acknowledging feelings and concerns; and facilitating the exploration of alternate or modified methods of sexual expression. (See pages 93–108.)

FUTURE IMPLICATIONS

A large number of research projects are being conducted to gain further understanding of all dimensions of SCI—the pathophysiology, the systemic and psychological effects, and the efficacy of various treatment modalities. With the increased knowledge gained from these studies it is hoped that existing management methods can be improved and new methods can be developed to prevent or reverse SCI damage, to more effectively prevent and treat systemic complications, to maximize functional abilities, and to facilitate psychological adjustment to the disability.

Rehabilitation nurses play a key role in all phases of SCI management by participating in these research projects, by integrating their knowledge and skills to provide optimum nursing care to individuals with SCI, and by providing these individuals with ongoing psychological support and education to assist them in regaining control of their lives.

REFERENCES

American Spinal Cord Injury Association. (1987). *Standards for neurological classification of spinal cord injury patients*. Chicago: American Spinal Cord Injury Association.

Block, R., and Basbaum, M. (Eds.). (1986). *Management of spinal cord injuries*. Baltimore: Williams and Wilkins.

Bell, J., and Hannon, K. (1986). Pathology involved in autonomic dysreflexia. *Journal of Neuroscience Nursing, 18*(2):86.

Buchanan, L., and Narvoczenski, D. (Eds.). (1987). *Spinal cord injury: Concepts and management approaches*. Baltimore: Williams and Wilkins.

Chadwick, A., and Oesting, H. (1989). Not for specialists only: Caring for patients with spinal cord injuries. *Nursing 89, 19*(11):52–56.

Chu, D., Ahn, J., Ragnarsson, K., and Helt, J. (1985). Deep venous thrombosis: Diagnosis in spinal cord injured patients. *Archives of Physical Medicine and Rehabilitation, 66*(6):365–368.

Corbet, B. (1985). National Resource Directory. *Newton, MA: National Spinal Cord Injury Association*.

Cyr, L. (1989). Sequelae of SCI after discharge from the initial rehabilitation program. *Rehabilitation Nursing, 14*(6):326–329.

Frye, B. (1986). A model of wellness-seeking behaviors in traumatic spinal cord injury victims. *Rehabilitation Nursing, 11*(5):6–7.

Killen, J. (1990). Role stabilization in families after spinal cord injury. *Rehabilitation Nursing, 15*(1):19–21.

Kirby, N. (1989). The individual with high quadriplegia. *Nursing Clinics of North America, 24*(1):179–191.

Lloyd, E., and Baker, F. (1986). An examination of variables in spinal cord injury patients with pressure sores. *Spinal Cord Injury Nursing, 3*(2):19.

Meyers, A. (1985). Rehospitalization and spinal cord injury: Cross sectional survey of adults living independently. *Archives of Physical Medicine, 66*:704–706.

Nelson, A. (1990). Patient's perspectives of a spinal cord injury unit. *SCI Nursing, 7*(3):44–63.

Persaud, D., and Stowe, K. (Eds.). (1987). *Spinal cord injury educational guidelines for professional nursing practice.* New York: American Association of Spinal Cord Injury Nurses.

Saltzman, R., and Melvin, J. (1986). Ventilatory compromise in spinal cord injury–A review. *Journal of American Paraplegia Society, 9*(1,2):6.

Stover, S. (1986). *Spinal cord injury: Facts and figures.* Birmingham: University of Alabama Press.

Thompson, S. (1988). Protocols for pressure ulcer interventions. *SCI Nursing, 5*(3):41–47.

Trieschmann, R. (1987). *Aging with a disability.* New York: Demos Publications.

Weingarden, S., Weingarden, D., and Belen, J. (1988). Fever and thromboembolic disease in acute spinal cord injury. *Paraplegia, 26*:35–42.

Whiteneck, G., Adler, C., Carter, R., Lammertse, D., Manley, S., Menter, R., Wagner, K., and Wilmot, C. (1989). *The management of high quadriplegia.* New York: Demos Publications.

Cerebral Vascular Accident Management 10

OBJECTIVES

After completing this chapter, the reader will be able to:

- Identify the risk factors of stroke and discuss preventive interventions.
- Compare the etiologies of stroke in relation to onset and prognosis.
- Correlate the clinical manifestations of stroke with the areas of brain damage.
- Discuss the differences in emotional/behavioral manifestations between a person with a right cerebral vascular accident (CVA) and one with a left CVA.
- Discuss the differences in perceptual spatial manifestations between the person with a right CVA and one with a left CVA.
- Discuss the potential musculoskeletal complications of a stroke and the appropriate preventive measures.
- Describe three intervention measures to assist the patient with perceptual spatial problems.
- Compare the teaching methods that would be used for a patient with a right CVA and one with a left CVA.

INTRODUCTION

CVA, or stroke, is one of the most frequently occurring neurological disorders. Each year over 500,000 people in the United States have strokes. Stroke-related mortality rises sharply with age and is near 50 percent in people who have strokes after the age of 70 and in those with pre-existing cerebrovascular disease, coma, or marked neurological deficit. Of those who survive the first attack, 20 percent suffer another stroke within the next 12 to 24 months.

In spite of these sobering statistics, data from several sources demonstrate up to a 45 percent decline in stroke incidence and mortality over the past 25 years. The decline was most evident in ischemic stroke and for intracerebral hemorrhage. Several factors may be contributing to this decline—the Surgeon General's warning on the hazards of smoking, the American Heart Association's recommendations for decreased intake of dietary fat and cholesterol, and improvements in hypertension detection and control.

Certain groups remain at higher risk for having a stroke. For example, 60 to 75 percent of strokes occur in people over the age of 65 years. Men are affected slightly more often than women and there is a higher incidence in the black population. Other stroke risk factors include hypertension, diabetes mellitus, heart disease (left ventricular hypertrophy, coronary artery disease, congestive heart failure, rheumatic heart disease and atrial fibrillation, and atrial fibrillation alone), polycythemia vera, hyperlipidemia, obesity, and smoking.

Rehabilitation nurses have a major role in all aspects of stroke management: Minimizing risk factors, preventing complications, providing preventive and self-care teaching, minimizing limitations, maximizing functional potential, and providing psychological support for the patient and family.

PATHOPHYSIOLOGY

An ischemic (thrombotic or embolic) stroke results from decreased blood flow to the brain secondary to a partial or complete occlusion of the artery. It occurs more frequently than a hemorrhagic stroke. Thrombus formation is the most common cause of an ischemic stroke. A thrombus is usually caused by atherosclerotic disease where plaques form in the arterial walls, precipitate platelet aggregation, thrombus formation, and vessel occlusion. Two-thirds of thrombotic strokes are associated with hypertension or diabetes mellitus. A thrombus can also develop from inflammatory vessel disorders such as syphilis, tuberculosis, and arteritis, as well as from cranial trauma.

A thrombotic stroke may be characterized by prodromal warnings (transient ischemic attacks and intermittent or erratic progression of neurological symptoms). Manifestations usually peak within 72 hours. The degree of neurological involvement depends on the rapidity of onset, size of lesion, and the presence of collateral circulation. As cerebral edema subsides some improvement is apparent within 2 weeks. Maximum improvement is usually attained within 12 to 24 weeks, though some functional changes may occur up to 2 years after onset. Recovery depends on the extent of the neurological damage, the area of brain involvement, and the presence of coexisting health problems. The more rapid the return of neurological function, the better the prognosis.

Embolism is the second most common cause of ischemic stroke. About 50 percent of embolic strokes originate in the endocardial layer of the heart with clots breaking off and entering the circulation. Contributing diseases include chronic atrial fibrillation (AF), myocardial infarction, and rheumatic heart disease with valve replacement. Other types of coronary pathology that cause AF, such as hypertensive, congenital, or syphilitic heart disease, can also lead to embolic strokes. The onset is usually sudden and unrelated to activity. Recurrence is common.

The amount of cerebral tissue damage and the degree of neurological recovery depends on the size of the embolus and the vessel affected. The destructive process begins when an embolus becomes lodged in a blood vessel. Then, in addition to the embolus, fibrous material from the vessel wall and clotting factors form plaques that lead to vessel occlusion. Edema and necrosis develop in the area supplied by the vessel.

Hemorrhagic strokes occur as a result of bleeding into either brain tissue or into the subarachnoid space. Intracerebral hemorrhage (ICH) accounts for about 10 to 20 percent of CVAs. ICH can occur spontaneously, usually as a result of hypertensive vascular disease which causes thickening, degeneration, and eventual rupture of the small cerebral arteries and subsequent hemorrhage or as a result of an arteriovenous malformation or following a carotid endarterectomy. Symptoms evolve over 1 to 2 hours and include headache, nausea and vomiting, and decreased responsiveness. The prognosis for survival is worse than for an ischemic stroke as the damage is usually more extensive. Survival and the degree of neurological recovery is related to the extent and location of the hemorrhage. The average mortality rate for ICH is about 50 percent.

An aneurysm rupture is the most frequent cause of subarachnoid hemorrhage (SAH). It usually occurs with an activity such as straining or lifting. It may also occur following trauma. One third occur during sleep. The first symptoms are usually severe headache and nuchal rigidity. A rapidly elevating intracranial pressure can lead to subsequent herniation and death. The mortality rate for SAH is about 45 percent. Recurrence of bleeds occurs in about one-third of the survivors. If a person does survive the initial and subsequent bleeds, the prognosis for neurological recovery is better than for an ischemic stroke. Table 10-1 summarizes the treatment approaches for ischemic and hemorrhagic strokes.

Classification

Ischemic events are described according to the temporal course and eventual outcome. Transient ischemic attacks (TIAs) are episodes of temporary focal dysfunction of vascular origin. The onset is rapid (usually less than 5 minutes) and the duration is variable (usually 2 to 15 minutes). By definition no neurological deficit remains after the attack. Transient symptoms vary according to the area of ischemia. Unilateral symptoms predominate with carotid system ischemia (unilateral weakness and sensory complaints, unilateral facial paresis or paresthesia, amaurosis fugax, dysphagia) compared to bilateral symptoms with vertebrobasilar ischemia (bilateral motor and sensory deficits, binocular visual complaints, ataxia, dysarthria, dysphasia, diplopia, vertigo, nausea, vomiting). The primary cause of TIA is a microembolism to the brain from atherosclerotic plaques in the cranial arteries. Other causes include emboli associated with valvular disease of the heart, polycythemia vera, and other blood clotting disorders. TIA is an important warning sign of an impending stroke as 25 to 35 percent of TIA victims later have strokes.

With a reversible ischemic neurological deficit (RIND), neurological symptoms may last from 24 hours to 2 weeks. There is no residual damage after 2 weeks. RIND episodes are similar to TIAs in symptomology, pathogenesis, and treatment. Stroke in evolution (SIE) refers to a condition of stroke progression and deteriorating neurological function over a period of several hours or as long as 2 to 3 days. The cause is usually from an arterial thrombosis. With a

TABLE 10-1 Medical Treatments for CVA

Condition	Treatment
Thrombotic Stroke/ low flow states	Reduce brain damage by maintaining adequate perfusion and by reducing edema formation during acute phase. Antiplatelet therapy (aspirin most effective). Anticoagulation for SIE. Blood pressure control and avoidance of overtreatment. Blood glucose control. Calcium channel blockers. Hypovolemic hemodilution. Surgery to augment blood flow.
Embolic Stroke	Reduce brain damage by maintaining adequate perfusion and by reducing edema formation during acute phase. Blood pressure control. Blood glucose control. Anticoagulation. Administration of clot dissolving agents. Surgery to remove embolic source.
Hemorrhagic Stroke	Reduce brain damage by maintaining adequate perfusion and by reducing edema formation during acute phase. Blood pressure control. Prevention of complications of autonomic discharge, hypovolemia, electrolyte imbalance, elevated ICP, hypoxia, recurrent hemorrhage. Surgical repair of site if feasible.

completed stroke (CS) the maximum neurological deficit has been acquired and the patient's condition is usually stable or improving. The onset is likely to be sudden when the infarct is caused by an embolus or hemorrhage and slower (SIE) when caused by an arterial thrombosis.

Impairments Related to Area of Damage

The type and extent of impairments resulting from a stroke depend on the site and size of the damaged area of the brain. These impairments include motor deficits (plegia or paresis, dysphagia,

TABLE 10-2 Potential Impairments Following CVA: A Comparison by Hemispheres

Left CVA	Right CVA

1. Sensory motor
  a. Right hemiplegia/paresis
  b. Spasticity
  c. Impaired balance, coordination
  d. Right side paresthesias
	1. Sensory motor
	  a. Left hemiplegia/paresis
	  b. Spasticity
	  c. Impaired balance, coordination
	  d. Left side paresthesias

2. Vision
  a. Right homonymous hemianopsia
  b. Field cut
  c. Impaired depth perception
	2. Vision
	  a. Left homonymous hemianopsia
	  b. Field cut
	  c. Impaired depth perception
	  d. Impaired facial recognition

3. Communication
  a. Aphasia
    (1) Nonfluent, Broca's expressive
    (2) Fluent, Wernicke's, receptive
  b. Dysarthria
	3. Communication
	  a. Very talkative
	
	  b. Dysarthria

4. Swallowing
  a. Dysphagia
	4. Swallowing
	  a. Dysphagia

5. Emotional/behavioral
  a. Lability
  b. Overcaution
  c. Anxiety
  d. Low frustration tolerance
  e. Depression
	5. Emotional/behavioral
	  a. Lability
	  b. Impulsivity
	  c. Overconfidence
	  d. Carelessness
	  e. Distractability

6. Perceptual spatial
  a. Apraxia
  b. Impaired right-left
  . discrimination
	6. Perceptual spatial
	  a. Apraxia
	  b. Anosognosia
	  c. Gets lost easily

6. Fatigue	6. Fatigue

7. Cognition
  a. Attention, memory, reasoning, abstraction, generalization, problem-solving, and judgment deficits
	7. Cognition
	  a. Attention, memory, reasoning, abstraction, generalization, problem-solving, and judgment deficits

dysarthria), sensory (perceptual) deficits, language deficits (dysphasia), visual deficits (defects in the visual fields, visual agnosia, and diplopia), cognitive deficits, behavioral changes, and bowel and bladder dysfunction. Other specific impairments depend on the site of the occlusion and which hemisphere of the brain is involved. Table 10-2 provides a comparison of residual impairments by hemispheres.

Experimental Therapies

The following experimental therapies are being used in various medical centers to treat ischemic strokes. The results to date are encouraging though the statistics are limited.

With larger or superficial lesions and ischemia of recent onset, cerebral blood flow may be restored by dissolving clots with agents such as urokinase. This procedure needs to be initiated within 4 hours of symptom onset.

For occlusions of longer duration, a chemical blockade of intracellular ischemic changes can be initiated with a calcium channel blocker. This procedure needs to be initiated within 12 hours of symptom onset.

Hypovolemic hemodilution attempts to reduce the zone of oligemia surrounding an ischemic core by maximizing intravascular volume and optimizing the hematocrit to insure a maximum amount of oxygen delivery. This procedure needs to be initiated within 24 hours of symptom onset.

Other investigational agents that may be effective in reversing neurological impairment following acute stroke include thromboxane-synthetase inhibitors, platelet inhibitors, and opiate antagonists.

NURSING INTERVENTIONS

Assessment

Health History

Presence of risk factors: Hypertension, atherosclerosis, diabetes mellitus, cardiac disease, polycythemia vera, TIAs, head trauma, advanced age, family history of cardiovascular disease, tobacco use, stress, sedentary lifestyle, obesity, elevated fat and cholesterol levels, and birth control pill use.

- Other pre-existing conditions or diseases.
- Pattern of stroke progression.
- Current medications.
- Known allergies.
- History of seizures.
- Personal history including diet, sleep, smoking, and exercise pattern and psychosocial status.

Physical Assessment Findings

- Vital sign instability, presence of headache, nausea, vomiting, vertigo.
- Behavior disturbances evidenced by impulsivity, depression, anxiety.
- Motor dysfunction evidenced by plegia, paresis, spasticity, hypotonia/flaccidity, ataxia, pathological reflexes.
- Absent or diminished response to touch, pain, pressure, heat, cold, position.
- Perceptual deficits evidenced by anosognosia, neglect, impaired right left discrimination, temporal disorientation, apraxias, agnosias.
- Cranial nerve dysfunction evidenced by dysphagia, diplopia, dysarthria.
- Cognitive dysfunction evidenced by impaired abilities of attention, memory, abstraction, reasoning, generalization, problem-solving, executive function, judgment.
- Communication deficits evidenced by impaired written and verbal comprehension and output.

Diagnostic Tests

- Computed tomography (CT scan) to show size and location of lesion, to differentiate infarction and hemorrhage, and to determine course of healing.
- Nuclear magnetic resonance imaging (NMR) to visualize brain structures and associated changes.
- Positron emission tomography (PET scan) to demonstrate chemical activity in brain and show extent of tissue damage.

- Electroencephalogram (EEG) to show abnormal electrical activity in brain.
- Arteriogram to show thrombus and vascular narrowing and to identify collateral blood supply, aneurysm, or arteriovenous malformation.
- Digital intravenous angiography (DIVA) to show distortion of cerebral vascular system.
- Lumbar puncture to show blood in cerebrospinal fluid and/or elevated pressure, to detect infection or other possible nonvascular causes of symptoms.
- Iodine radionucleotide brain scan to differentiate between CVA and non-vascular conditions.
- Doppler to evaluate carotid circulation.
- Risk factor tests including lipid profiles and hypertension workup.

Nursing Diagnoses: Actual or Potential

1. Impaired cognition related to attention, memory, abstract reasoning, generalization, problem solving, executive function, and judgment deficits.
2. Impaired physical mobility related to paresis, plegia, spasticity, decreased endurance.
3. Impaired communication related to aphasia, dysarthria, dyslexia, dysgraphia.
4. Sensory perceptual alterations: Visual, auditory, kinesthetic, tactile related to altered sensory reception, transmission and/or integration.
5. Potential for injury related to sensory, motor, and/or cognitive deficits, seizures.
6. Self-care deficits related to motor, sensory, and/or cognitive deficits, fatigue, depression.
7. Activity intolerance related to motor deficits, deconditioning, and fatigue.
8. Altered tissue perfusion: Cerebral related to impaired arterial circulation to brain.
9. Respiratory dysfunction: Hypoventilation related to respiratory muscle weakness; pulmonary congestion related to aspiration or immobility.
10. Impaired skin integrity related to immobility, sensory and

cognitive deficits, mechanical factors, altered nutritional status, impaired circulation.

11. Altered bowel elimination: Constipation related to immobility, lack of privacy, inadequate diet and fluid intake; diarrhea related to tube feedings.
12. Altered nutritional status: Less than body requirements related to chewing/swallowing difficulties, inability to feed self.
13. Uncompensated swallowing impairment related to neurological dysfunction.
14. Altered urinary elimination: Incontinence related to cognitive and motor deficits.
15. Sexual dysfunction related to biopsychosocial alteration of sexuality, fatigue, absence of role models, lack of privacy, lack of knowledge.
16. Social isolation related to sensory, motor, and cognitive deficits; self-concept disturbances.
17. Disturbance in self-concept: Body image, self-esteem.
18. Anxiety related to threat to self-concept, role functioning and interaction patterns; unmet needs.
19. Grieving: Dysfunctional or anticipatory related to actual or perceived losses.
20. Ineffective individual or family coping related to inadequate information, inadequate support, multiple life changes.
21. Knowledge deficit related to CVA management.

Expected Outcomes: Patient and/or Family

1. The individual demonstrates improved cognitive abilities.
2. The individual maintains functional alignment and sustains no complications of immobility.
3. The individual uses correct techniques to facilitate mobility and to compensate for motor, sensory, and cognitive deficits.
4. The individual's program is planned to provide adequate rest periods.
5. The individual is comfortable as evidenced by verbal statements and/or body language.
6. The individual employs an effective method of communication to convey thoughts and needs.
7. The individual re-establishes role functions and socialization

patterns and engages in self-care activities consistent with sensory, motor, and/or cognitive limitations.

8. The individual remains free of injury.
9. The individual's lungs remain clear.
10. The individual's skin integrity is restored or maintained.
11. The individual's bladder and bowel patterns are stabilized.
12. The individual is free of bowel and bladder complications.
13. The individual maintains nutritional status as evidenced by stable body weight and normal hemoglobin, hematocrit, and serum protein.
14. The individual verbalizes perception of himself/herself as a sexual being.
15. The individual experiences decreased anxiety and improved self-concept as evidenced by verbal statements and/or body language.
16. The individual verbalizes and demonstrates an understanding of CVA management.

Planning and Implementation

(Include the family, significant other, and/or caregiver in the teaching interventions.)

Risk Management

Facilitate prevention measures by teaching the patient how to control risk factors through low fat, low cholesterol diet, weight control, stress management, elimination of tobacco use, adherence to treatment regimes for hypertension, diabetes mellitus, and other vascular diseases, and recognition of stroke warning signs.

Systemic Management

If the stroke is in evolution, place the patient at rest in a calm, non-stimulating environment. Reduce anxiety by providing information, allowing ventilation of feelings, and permitting the family to remain.

If the CVA is a thrombotic or embolic stroke, administer anticoagulants as ordered. Observe and record the patient's response. Take precautions to minimize side effects of the medication.

If the CVA is from a hypertensive bleed, administer antihypertensive medications as ordered. Observe and record the patient's response. Watch for signs of ischemia (increasing neurological deficits that can result from reducing blood pressure in diseased cerebral vessels).

If the CVA is from a ruptured or leaking aneurysm or arteriovenous malformation, administer antifibrinolytic medication as ordered. Observe and record the patient's response. Take precautions to minimize side effects of the medication.

Assist the patient to maximize functional potential, minimize spasticity, and prevent contractures. (See pages 148 and 150–151.) Bobath's neurodevelopmental therapy helps control patterns of spasticity by inhibiting abnormal reflex patterns and promoting bilateral functioning. Assist the patient in learning proper positioning, exercises, activities of daily living, and safety techniques.

Implement measures to prevent DVT, PE, and respiratory complications related to immobility and paralysis. Assist the patient in learning preventive measures. (See pages 143–144.)

Implement measures to prevent skin breakdown related to immobility, sensory deficits, nutritional deficits, and incontinence. Assist the patient in learning preventive measures. (See pages 146–148.)

Maintain adequate fluid intake and nutrition by monitoring the patient's weight, calorie and fluid intake, and serum protein levels, working with the nutritionist to provide a high protein balanced diet according to the patient's preferences, and working with the occupational therapist to provide adaptive eating aids as needed. Minimize patient fatigue by providing small, more frequent feedings. Provide mouth care after each meal to make sure no food is still in the mouth that could be aspirated. Assist the patient in learning proper food selection, fluid and nutritional requirements, and on safe eating/feeding techniques.

If dysphagia is present, implement the appropriate management and teaching program. (See pages 81–92.)

Implement a bowel management program to prevent constipation related to immobility, dehydration, and inadequate diet. Assist the patient in learning prevention and problem resolution management. (See pages 69–80.)

Implement a bladder management program to prevent incontinence, calculi, and infection related to neurogenic dysfunction, immobility, and dehydration. Assist the patient in learning prevention and treatment measures. (See pages 51–68.)

Provide frequent scheduled rest periods to help the patient cope with the fatigue related to the brain damage and recovery process. (Without proper management fatigue can temporarily exacerbate cognitive, behavioral, and physical problems.

Cognitive Management

(Refer to pages 123–125 for further information related to cognitive management.)

To facilitate expressive and receptive communication skills, work with the speech pathologist on a program individualized for the patient. Speak slowly in a normal voice. Use short simple sentences. Periodically assess comprehension. Be patient and avoid overcorrecting or interrupting. Minimize distractions without isolating the individual. Encourage family members and others to stay close and within the patient's line of vision during communication exchanges. Provide frequent positive feedback to the individual. Use nonverbal modalities such as demonstrations to facilitate comprehension. Monitor environmental factors.

For impaired attention avoid overstimulation. Simplify the environment and limit distractions. Maintain consistent one-to-one interactions. Provide simple, concrete, repetitive instructions and eliminate extraneous stimuli. Provide structured situations that attach meaning to input and keep sessions brief. Assess for pain, fatigue, and other possible causes of distractibility.

For impaired memory system, reasoning, abstraction, and generalization abilities, provide structure, consistency, and repetition. Emphasize old, over-learned, familiar skills. Use multiple modalities for teaching (auditory, visual, tactile) but keep approach structured and consistent. Pair old, familiar information with the new. Teach in a situational environment. Use memory aids and techniques such as calendars, categorization, and pairing. Place daily activities in predictable, step by step sequence. Start with simple tasks in a structured format then build complexity and gradually decrease structure.

For problem solving and executive function deficits, assist the patient in developing short-term, achievable goals; participating in the planning process; and following through with each step of the plan. Assist the patient in evaluating his/her progress and in making necessary modifications in the plan.

For impaired insight and judgment assist the patient in understanding the concept of brain damage and how it has affected him/

her physically, cognitively, and emotionally. Encourage him/her to participate in peer group programs for sharing feelings, identifying problems, and working out solutions through group feedback.

Assist the family in understanding the patient's cognitive problems and in learning how to effectively assist him/her in coping with these problems.

Affective and Behavioral Management

Nearly one-half of the people who suffer strokes each year experience a full fledged bout of clinical depression. Depression in people with left CVAs is tied to decreases in the levels of serotonin. These depressions are usually more violent and catastrophic than right CVA depression, which is one of indifference and apathy. Decreased serotonin does not appear to play a role in right CVA depression. People with right hemisphere damage seem to be more susceptible to depression. A family history of depression increases the patient's risk of developing post stroke depression. The depression is most likely to start about 10 days after the stroke.

Work with the psychologist and other team members to create a therapy plan that addresses the patient's emotional state and needs. Refer the patient for individual or group counseling when appropriate. Administer antidepressive medications as prescribed. Observe and record the patient's response. Take precautions to minimize side effects of the medication. Avoid isolation and encourage interaction. Encourage the maintenance of an optimum nutrition program and a balanced rest and activity schedule.

For impulsivity teach methods of self-control with a simple reward system. Provide immediate but non-punitive feedback on inappropriate behavior. Redirect patient's attention to appropriate behavior.

Assist the patient in avoiding stress and fatigue that can exacerbate labile episodes. Avoid focusing on lability by shifting the patient's attention to an unrelated subject. Labile episodes will usually decrease or resolve as recovery progresses.

Assist the patient and family to understand and cope with behavioral changes by providing appropriate explanations and by encouraging them to ventilate their feelings.

Perceptual Spatial Management

To help the patient compensate for neglect, impaired sensation, and proprioceptive problems, give frequent verbal, visual, and tactile cues to encourage awareness of the affected body parts. Encourage him/her to use feedback from the other senses. Protect affected body parts from injury and place the affected arm in a position to enhance visual awareness. Maintain a safe, well-lighted, uncluttered environment.

For spatial/perceptual deficits and apraxias divide tasks into simple, sequential steps and provide step-by-step guidance as needed. Allow for sufficient time to complete tasks. For nonaphasic patients use descriptive words and avoid spatial concepts when giving directions. Modify the environment to maximize performance by having personal care items and other aids accessible to the patient and by removing obstructive furniture.

To help the patient compensate for homonomous hemianopsia and prevent injury, teach scanning techniques. Approach from the midline or unaffected side. Place food and needed items in the unaffected visual field to lessen frustration; place them in the affected visual field to enhance compensation. Maintain a safe, well-lighted environment.

For visual midline displacement instruct the patient to lean the other way. Observe safety precautions in wheelchair positioning and with ambulation.

For visual vertical horizontal problems encourage the patient to use full-length mirrors and other senses for feedback.

For right left discrimination problems color code or label clothes. Use terms such as strong and weak side rather than right and left.

For altered time perception refer to time concepts in terms of activity rather than minutes and hours. Clocks usually do not help with altered time perception.

Assist the family in understanding the patient's perceptual deficits and in learning how to provide appropriate assistance while facilitating his/her independence. Reinforce safety awareness with the patient and family.

FUTURE IMPLICATIONS

The safety, self care, and emotional problems encountered by persons with strokes are often exacerbated through inappropriate interventions. Lack of time and ability can limit the accuracy of perceptual evaluations made by the rehabilitation team. Without proper identification of their specific deficits, patients may never achieve their full functional potentials, or they may do so only after many misguided and frustrating attempts. They are also more likely to have frequent falls and other preventable mishaps. Studies indicate that nearly 40 percent of the stroke population that experiences depression is not adequately diagnosed and treated, a therapeutic shortcoming that can lengthen depressive episodes by many months.

Despite these and other diagnostic and treatment shortcomings, significant progress continues in the area of stroke rehabilitation. Diagnostic techniques are becoming more sophisticated and accurate, which facilitates earlier, more constructive medical intervention. An expanded understanding of stroke pathophysiology is contributing to the development of medications that can prevent a stroke or reduce the cerebral ischemic damage if one does occur. In addition, advances in speech, cognitive, and behavioral therapies have the potential to increase each person's functional potential and enhance his/her quality of life.

REFERENCES

Baggerly, J. (1987). Impaired neurological functioning. In Rehabilitation Nursing Foundation. *Application of Rehabilitation Concepts to Nursing Practice.* Evanston: Rehabilitation Nursing Foundation.

Boss, B. (1988). The nervous system. In Howe, J., Dickason, E., Jones, D., and Snider, M. (Eds.). *The handbook of nursing.* New York: John Wiley and Sons, Inc.

Dudas, L. (1986). Nursing diagnoses and interventions for the rehabilitation of the stroke patient. *Nursing Clinics of North America, 21*(2):345–357.

Gee, Z., and Passarella, P. (1985). *Nursing care of the stroke patient: A therapeutic approach.* Pittsburgh: American Rehabilitation Educational Network.

Hickey, J. (1986). *The clinical practice of neurological and neurosurgical nursing* (2nd ed.). Philadelphia: J. B. Lippincott Company.

Kaplan, P. (1986). Stroke and rehabilitation. In Brody, S., and Ruft, G. (Eds.). *Age and rehabilitation.* New York: Springer Publishing Company.

Kelly, J., and Winograd, C. (1985). A functional approach to stroke management in elderly patients. *Journal of American Geriatric Society, 33*:48–60.

Lewis, N. (1986). Functional gains in CVA patients: Nursing approaches. *Rehabilitation Nursing, 11*(2):25–27.

Marshall, S., Marshall, L., Vos, H., and Randall, C. (1990). *Neuroscience critical care: Pathophysiology and patient management.* Philadelphia: W. B. Saunders.

Millikan, C., McDowell, F., and Easton, J. (1987). *Stroke.* Philadelphia: Lea and Febiger.

Mumma, C. (1986). Perceived losses following stroke. *Rehabilitation Nursing, 11*(3):19–24.

Mumma, C. (1987). Stroke patient. In Lewis, S., and Collier, I. *Medical surgical nursing: Assessment and management of clinical problems* (2nd ed.). New York: McGraw Hill Book Company.

Ozuna, J. (1987). Chronic neurological conditions. In Lewis, S., and Collier, I. (Eds.). *Medical surgical nursing: Assessment and management of clinical problems.* New York: McGraw Hill Book Company.

Passarella, P., and Gee, Z. (1987). Starting right after stroke. *American Journal of Nursing, 87*(6):802–807.

Pierce, L. (1988). Stroke support group: A reality. *Rehabilitation Nursing, 13*(4):189–190.

Plum, F., and Pulsinelli, W. (1985). *Cerebrovascular disease.* New York: Raven Press.

Quandt, C., Talbert, R., and De Los Reyes, R. (1987). Current concepts in clinical therapeutics: Ischemic cerebrovascular disease. *Clinical Pharmacy, 6*(4):292–306.

Sindor, D., et al. (1986). Post-stroke depression: Relationships and functional impairment, coping strategies, and rehabilitation outcomes. *Stroke, 17*(6):1102–1106.

Tanner, D., Gerstenberger, D., and Keller, C. (1989). Guidelines for treatment of chronic depression in the aphasic patient. *Rehabilitation Nursing, 14*(2):77–80, 87.

Taylor, J. (1985). Nursing management of stroke: Acute care–Part II. *Cardiovascular Nursing, 21*(2):7–12.

Multiple Sclerosis Management

11

OBJECTIVES

After completing this chapter, the reader will be able to:

- Describe the pathophysiology of multiple sclerosis (MS) and discuss the theories of etiology.
- Discuss methods to control potential exacerbating factors.
- Discuss the alterations in motor, sensory, and cognitive function associated with MS.
- Describe the respiratory, urological, and gastrointestinal complications that may develop with MS and discuss preventive and treatment measures.
- Discuss interventions for maximizing the patient's functional potential.
- Discuss interventions for enhancing the patient's coping skills and facilitating psychosocial adjustment.

INTRODUCTION

MS affects an estimated 500,000 people in the United States, with females affected slightly more frequently than males. The onset of symptoms usually occurs between the ages of 20 and 40. The degree of physical impairment depends on the stage and severity of the disease and can range from no observable deficits to total disability. Because of the highly variable patterns persons with MS must live with the ongoing anxiety and uncertainty of how the disease will manifest itself over time and how it will impact on their lives. The rehabilitation nurse and other members of the rehabilitation team must provide ongoing psychological support along with a well-coordinated therapy and educational program to help these individuals maximize their abilities, cope with the uncertainties, and prepare for the future.

PATHOPHYSIOLOGY

MS, or disseminated sclerosis, is a chronic progressive degenerative disease of the central nervous system (CNS). An agent of unknown etiology produces scattered patches of inflammation in the myelin sheath covering the nerve fibers in the brain and spinal cord. The accompanying impairment of motor, sensory, and cognitive functions are initially due to failure of the nerve fibers to effectively conduct impulses across these lesions because of edema-related pressure in the acute phase or from myelin damage in the chronic phase. Later, permanent functional losses are caused by scar formation (sclerotic plaques) in old lesions and destruction of nerve fibers.

The course of the disease is highly variable. Initially, a period of exacerbation may be followed by an extended remission with no evidence of symptoms. This apparent recovery is attributed to a resolution of the inflammatory process and a partial remyelination, or healing, of the damaged myelin. With repeated attacks the scarring becomes more extensive and ultimately the nerve fibers become damaged. Many researchers believe that the pattern established in the first 3 years following diagnosis may be an indicator of what the person can expect in the future. Table 11-1 describes the patterns most frequently encountered in various forms of MS.

Etiology Theories

The etiology of MS is unknown; however, many studies are being conducted in an attempt to identify the causative factors and the factors that may influence susceptibility. One possible influence on susceptibility appears to be geography. MS is more prevalent in the northern latitudes of the world where the incidence is 30 to 800 per 100,000. In the temperate zones the incidence of MS is 1 per 100,000. Another possible influence on susceptibility seems to be genetic. The incidence of MS is 15 times higher in families that al-

TABLE 11-1 Types of Multiple Sclerosis

Type	Characteristics
Benign	Few, mild, early exacerbations and complete or nearly complete remissions. Minimal or no disability. About 20% of the cases.
Exacerbating-Remitting	More frequent, early exacerbation with less complete remissions. Long periods of stability with some degree of disability. About 25% of the cases.
Chronic-Relapsing	Fewer and less complete remissions. Cumulative disability ranging from moderate to severe. About 40% of the cases.
Chronic-Progressive	Slowly progressive with no remissions. Cumulative disability ranging from moderate to severe. About 15% of the cases.

ready have one family member with the disease. The exact mechanisms related to the geographic and genetic correlations are unknown at this time.

Several causation theories are currently under investigation. One of these theories proposes that common viruses such as those causing measles, chicken pox, and upper respiratory infections may trigger a delayed auto-immune response, which causes the body's own defense system to attack the myelin sheath resulting in inflammation, edema, myelin and nerve fiber destruction and scarring. Another viral causation theory proposes that there may be a MS specific slow-acting virus that causes the myelin damage. At this time no specific viruses have been identified. Another theory suggests that toxin exposure may play a role initiating or perpetuating the destructive process. No direct link has been made with any specific toxin at this time.

Some of the factors associated with the initial onset of symptoms or exacerbation of symptoms include infection, vaccinations, trauma, over-fatigue, exposure to extreme heat or cold, menses, pregnancy, and other physical and psychological stresses. Exacerbations are usually more common and more severe in the early stages of MS. An older person with MS usually experiences few at-tacks, suggesting that the body may develop some control over the disease process. The effects of pregnancy on the course of MS are controversial. Some studies report an increased incidence of exacer-bation in the first 3 months following delivery, but there is no evi-dence that this affects the long-term course of the disease.

Research

In addition to the etiological studies, many other research studies are being conducted. These studies focus on four primary goals.

One goal is to prevent further damage to the CNS by stopping the underlying disease process through the use of immunosuppressive drugs such as cyclophosphamide (Cytoxan) or azathioprine (Imuran) or through the use of a vaccine such as copolymer[1]; by eliminating inflammation through the use of adrenocorticotropic hormone (ACTH), high doses of steroid drugs such as methylprednisolone or with cyclosporine (Sandimmune), which is both immunosuppres-sive and anti-inflammatory; and by preventing the development of scarring through the blockage of astrocyte (CNS cells which pro-duce scarring) stimulation.

A second goal is to reverse the damage already done by restoring myelin in MS lesions through oligodendrocyte (the cells which make and maintain myelin) stimulation with injections of certain myelin components; by promoting a regrowth of damaged nerve fibers; and by reducing existing scars.

A third goal is to improve function in MS patients by restoring conduction in nonfunctioning nerve fibers with medication such as 4-aminopyridine; by reducing spasticity with drugs currently in use such as baclophen (Lioresal) and with others being tested such as ti-zanidine, progabide, ketazolam, and thyrotropin-releasing hormone.

A fourth goal is to provide more accurate and complete prognos-tic information with additional findings from current genetic re-search and immunological tests, with the use of neuro-imaging stud-ies, and with cognitive and psychological testing.

Classification

The onset of symptoms of MS may appear slowly over a period of weeks or months, or it may begin suddenly and dramatically. One

TABLE 11-2 Classification of Primary Lesion Sites

Lesion Site	Related Impairments/Symptoms
Spinal Cord	Motor: Paresis or paralysis, incoordination, tremor, spasticity, hyperactive reflexes. Sensory: Paresthesias, pain. Bladder: Urgency, frequency, incontinence, retention. Bowel: Constipation. Sexual: Impotency, ejaculatory dysfunction.
Cerebral	Cognitive: Impaired memory, impaired abstraction and reasoning, impaired judgment and problem solving.
Brain Stem	Vertigo, nausea, cranial nerves: Diplopia, tinnitus, dysphagia.
Cerebellum	Ataxia, intention tremor, instability, incoordination.
Mixed	Early in the disease almost all cases can be classified in one of the previous categories. However, after about 15 years most patients demonstrate a mixed involvement.

means of classifying the variety of MS presentations is according to the predominant site of the lesions (Table 11-2). The disabling symptoms of MS are classified in three categories: Primary (resulting directly from the MS lesions in the CNS as seen in Table 11-2); secondary (complicating conditions such as urinary tract infection and calculi, pneumonia, contractures, and decubiti); and tertiary (emotional, social, marital, economic, and vocational issues related to the disease).

Fatigue is a primary symptom. Though it doesn't result directly from CNS lesions, it does occur as a result of the pathophysiology of the disease. Extreme sensitivity to temperature changes is also related to the pathophysiology of the disease and can further exacerbate some of the primary symptoms; nerve conduction slows down as body temperature rises.

Evaluation and Documentation Tools

The minimal record of disability (MRD) is an evaluation and documentation tool developed by the International Federation of MS Societies. It organizes neurological, functional, psychological, and demographic information to provide a standardized method of communicating current, objective information on the individual with MS. The Functional Model (FM) incorporates data from the MRD plus information gathered by the patient. It is a useful tool for identifying the individual's strengths and weaknesses, setting goals, determining the associated education needs, and documenting the progress toward achieving the goals. Abilities are categorized in five levels: Functional/independent, functional with adaptation, functional with mechanical assistance, functional with mechanical and human assistance, and functionally dependent. The ultimate purpose of the FM is to move away from a negative, problem-focused treatment approach and provide a positive focus with emphasis on strengths instead of weaknesses, health; instead of illness, and ability instead of disability.

The Kurtzke rating method is another tool used to document and communicate the impairment level of MS patients. It is comprised of the functional systems (FS) with eight categories that summarize various components of the neurological examination and the mobility scale which assigns a score related to the degree of independence in function. The FS scores are integrated with the mobility score to obtain a global rating of neurological impairment, the expanded disability status scale (EDSS).

NURSING INTERVENTIONS

Assessment

Health History

- Complains of fatigue and lack of energy, frequently of weeks to months duration.
- Complains of heaviness, numbness, tingling in extremities and vague joint and muscle pains.
- Complains of vertigo.
- Complains of visual changes such as decreased acuity and diplopia.
- Complains of muscle weakness with foot dragging, falls, dropping objects; weakness worse after exposure to heat (Ulthoff's phenomena).
- Complains of constipation and urinary urgency or retention.
- Behavioral changes such as apathy, inattentiveness, depression, mood swings.
- Pre-existing conditions or diseases.

- Current medications.
- Known allergies.
- Personal history including diet, sleep, smoking, and exercise patterns and psychosocial status.

Physical Assessment Findings

- Motor dysfunction evidenced by muscle weakness, spasticity, hyperactive reflexes, positive Babinski's sign, ataxia, intention tremor, instability, uncoordination.
- Sensory changes evidenced by paresthesias, decreased temperature awareness, decreased vibration sense, loss of proprioception and joint sensation.
- Sensation of electric shock which extends down arms and back when neck is flexed (Lhermitte's sign).
- Visual changes evidenced by diplopia, loss of acuity, ophthalmoplegia of lateral gaze, central scotoma, visual field deficit, optic retrobulbar neuritis, nystagmus.
- Cognitive and behavioral changes evidenced by impaired memory, impaired abstraction and reasoning, impaired judgment and problem solving, lability, irritability.
- Speech impairments evidenced by spastic dysarthria, ataxic dysarthria with scanning speech, low volume.
- Bladder dysfunction evidenced by frequency, urgency, incontinence, or retention.

Diagnostic Tests

- Studies to rule out CNS tumors and/or to visualize plaques such as computed tomography (CT scan), positron emission tomography (PET scan), skull x-rays, myelogram, pneumogram, and magnetic resonance imaging (MRI).
- Evoked potential studies to reveal abnormal visual, auditory, and somatosensory responses.
- Cerebrospinal fluid (CSF) analysis to reveal an elevated level of gamma globulin to total protein.
- CSF immunoelectrophoretic assay to reveal elevated oligoclonal immunoglobulin G (IgG).

The diagnosis of MS is difficult to make because many of the symptoms present during an exacerbation may disappear during a remission. Therefore, the physician must look for suspicious patterns such as an exacerbation-remission cycle of neurological deficits, worsening of symptoms during and after exposure to heat, and a family history of MS. The final diagnosis is usually made only after all other possible causes of neuromuscular dysfunction have been ruled out, plaques have been visualized with neuro-imaging studies, and evoked potential studies have revealed abnormal visual, auditory, and somatosensory responses.

Nursing Diagnoses: Actual or Potential

1. Impaired cognition related to impaired memory, abstraction, reasoning, judgment, and problem solving abilities.
2. Impaired physical mobility related to paralysis, spasticity, pain, decreased endurance.
3. Altered comfort: Pain related to spasticity, immobility, and/or altered sensory responses.
4. Impaired communication related to motor, visual, and/or cognitive deficits.
5. Sensory perceptual alterations: Visual, kinesthetic, tactile related to altered sensory reception and transmission.
6. Potential for injury related to sensory, motor, and/or cognitive deficits.
7. Self-care deficits related to motor, sensory, and/or cognitive deficits, pain, fatigue.
8. Activity intolerance related to generalized weakness and fatigue.
9. Respiratory dysfunction: Hypoventilation related to respiratory muscle weakness; pulmonary congestion related to aspiration or immobility.
10. Impaired skin integrity related to immobility, sensory deficits, mechanical factors, altered nutritional status.
11. Altered bowel elimination: Constipation, incontinence related to immobility, neurological dysfunction, lack of privacy, inadequate diet.
12. Altered nutritional status: Less than body requirements related to anorexia, chewing/swallowing difficulties, inability to feed self.
13. Uncompensated swallowing impairment related to neurological dysfunction.

14. Altered urinary elimination: Incontinence, frequency, or retention related to neurological dysfunction.
15. Sexual dysfunction related to biopsychosocial alteration of sexuality, absence of role models, lack of privacy, lack of knowledge.
16. Social isolation related to sensory, motor, cognitive, and communication deficits.
17. Disturbance in self-concept: Body image, self-esteem.
18. Anxiety related to threat to self-concept, role functioning and interaction patterns; unmet needs.
19. Grieving: Dysfunctional or anticipatory related to actual or perceived losses.
20. Ineffective individual or family coping related to inadequate information, inadequate support, multiple life changes.
21. Knowledge deficit related to MS management.

Expected Outcomes: Patient and/or Family

1. The individual maintains cognitive abilities.
2. The individual maintains functional alignment and sustains no complications of immobility.
3. The individual uses correct techniques to facilitate mobility and to compensate for motor and sensory deficits.
4. The individual's activity program is planned to provide adequate rest periods.
5. The individual is comfortable as evidenced by verbal statements and/or body language.
6. The individual employs an effective method of communication to convey thoughts and needs.
7. The individual re-establishes role functions and socialization patterns and engages in self-care activities consistent with sensory, motor, and/or cognitive limitations.
8. The individual remains free of injury.
9. The individual's lungs remain clear.
10. The individual's skin integrity is restored or maintained.
11. The individual is free of urinary and bowel complications.
12. The individual's bowel and bladder patterns are stabilized.
13. The individual maintains nutritional status as evidenced by stable body weight and normal hemoglobin, hematocrit, and serum protein.

14. The individual verbalizes perception of himself/herself as a sexual being.
15. The individual experiences decreased anxiety and improved self-care concept as evidenced by verbal statements and/or body language.
16. The individual verbalizes and demonstrates an understanding of MS management.

Planning and Implementation

(Include the family, significant other, and/or caregiver in the teaching interventions.)

Neurological Management

General: Assist the patient in learning how to minimize or eliminate exacerbating factors of

(a) *Over-fatigue* by showing the patient how to use energy saving techniques, how to maintain a balanced schedule of rest and activity, and how to recognize the signals that indicate his/her endurance limit is approaching. When fatigue is associated with depression or anxiety, the patient may benefit from prescribed antidepressants such as trazodone (Desyrel) or from a mild stimulant such as pemoline (Cylert).
(b) *Overheating* by showing the patient the importance of avoiding overheated areas, hot baths and showers, and the use of hot water bottles and heating pads.
(c) and (d) *Infection* and *trauma* by showing the patient respiratory urological, and integumentary prevention techniques and safety techniques.
(e) *Psychological stresses* by assisting the patient in learning stress reduction strategies.

Reduce the severity of an exacerbation by administering medication as ordered (corticosteroids and/or adrenocorticotropic hormone) and by restricting strenuous activity during this time. Observe and record the patient's response. Take precautions to minimize side effects of the medication. Assist the patient in learning the medication purpose, dosage, schedule, side effects, and precautions.

Administer medications as ordered, such as the immunosuppressives azathioprine (Imuran) or cyclophosphamide (Cytoxan). Observe and record the patient's response. Take precautions to minimize side effects of the medication. Assist the patient in learning the medication purpose, dosage schedule, side effects, and precautions.

Administer medication as ordered, such as carbamazepine (Tegretol), phenytoin (Dilantin), or tricyclic antidepressants, to relieve painful hyperesthesias and nerve root pain. For low back pain and spasticity-related pain, administer antispasm, muscle relaxant, and/or analgesic medication as ordered. Observe and record the patient's response and take precautions to minimize side effects of the medication. Assist the patient in learning the medication purpose, dosage schedule, side effects, and precautions. Incorporate other pain management techniques appropriate to the type of pain, such as corrective positioning, supportive equipment, and transcutaneous nerve stimulation (TENS). Refer the patient for acupuncture or biofeedback when appropriate.

Assist the patient in learning about the pathophysiology, manifestations, and therapeutic management of MS.

Cognitive: Research studies indicate that after about 20 years, 25 percent of the severely disabled MS patients show varying degrees of cognitive deficits including impaired memory, abstraction, reasoning, judgment, and problem solving.

Implement measures that assist the patient to enhance cognitive functioning and minimize deficits; instruct the patient and family in these measures. (See pages 123–125.)

Visual: Assist the patient in learning how to compensate for visual impairment through the correct use of the appropriate aids such as an eye patch or frosted lens for diplopia, sunglasses to reduce glare sensitivity, and scanning for field cuts. Assist the patient in learning how to maintain a safe environment and monitor for hazards.

Speech: Work with the patient and the speech pathologist to improve the patient's compromised speech through exercises, positioning, modifications, postural devices, and fatigue prevention measures.

Respiratory Management

Implement measures to prevent respiratory complications. Assist the patient in learning preventive and treatment measures. (See pages 144–145.)

Cardiovascular Management

Implement measures to prevent deep vein thrombosis and pulmonary embolism. Assist the patient in learning preventive measures and symptom recognition. (See pages 143–144.)

Urological Management

Implement measures to manage urological dysfunction and prevent urological complications. Assist the patient in learning preventive and treatment measures. (See pages 51–68.)

Gastrointestinal Management

Implement a bowel management program to prevent constipation. Assist the patient in learning preventive and treatment measures. (See pages 69–80.)

Integumentary Management

Implement measures to prevent skin breakdown. Assist the patient in learning preventive and treatment measures. (See pages 146–148.)

Musculoskeletal Management

Gait dysfunction secondary to weakness, ataxia, spasticity, or a combination of these, is a major problem for the majority of persons with MS. Weakness and ataxia are not directly affected by interventions. However, consistent moderate exercise can prevent or reverse weakness caused by disuse and ambulation aids can facilitate mobility. Passive range of motion exercises help maintain joint mobility and prevent the development of contractures. Hydrotherapy facilitates movement and body heat is dissipated in the water.

Encourage the patient to walk with feet wider apart to increase walking stability. Caution the patient to avoid abrupt position changes.

Assist the patient in learning self-care techniques, maintenance and preventive exercises, safety measures, and the correct use of assistive equipment. Emphasize the importance of avoiding vigorous exercises as raised body temperature and fatigue can aggravate the patient's symptoms.

Implement prescribed measures to control spasticity. Assist the patient in learning preventive and treatment measures. (See pages 150–151.)

Psychological Management

To decrease anxiety and enhance coping skills, provide dependability and consistency in care. Eliminate or decrease environmental stressors as much as possible. Use a calm, unhurried approach when working with the patient. Structure the length and depth of interactions based on his/her needs and responses. Assist the patient and family to understand the stresses imposed by MS. Assist them in learning stress management techniques to more effectively handle these stresses.

To enhance self-esteem and minimize withdrawal, encourage the patient to keep up with social interests and activities. Provide positive feedback on learning and self-improvement efforts. Facilitate opportunities for peer interaction and sharing. Provide a referral to the National MS Society (205 East 42nd Street, New York, NY 10017-5706) and local groups for support and information. Assist the patient in understanding how to structure a daily activity schedule that will facilitate his/her successful completion of the activities with minimal stress and fatigue.

Refer the patient for psychological therapy as needed to assist him/her in dealing with depression and anxiety.

Sexuality Counseling

Assist the individual to maintain his/her sexual identity by minimizing the number of embarrassing, intrusive procedures and exposures, supporting the maintenance of physical appearance, acknowledging feelings and concerns, and facilitating the exploration of alternate or modified methods of sexual expression. (See pages 93–108.)

FUTURE IMPLICATIONS

There are many questions under investigation, and without definitive answers, regarding the etiology of MS, effective methods to prevent or reverse neurological damage, the most reliable prognostic indicators, and the most effective management techniques. Because of these many uncertainties, MS patients are faced with not only the stresses and challenges of their disability but with the stresses of dealing with a fluctuating and erratic disease course. Psychological support and education are key responsibilities for the rehabilitation nurse working with persons with MS and their families. By being informed consumers, they are less likely to be misled by the many erroneous, costly, and potentially hazardous claims that are constantly appearing in the lay magazines and papers. In addition they can regain a sense of control over the disease and their lives.

REFERENCES

Francabandera, F., Holland, N., Wiesel-Levinson, P., and Scheinberg, L. (1988). Multiple sclerosis rehabilitation: Inpatient vs. outpatient. *Rehabilitation Nursing, 13*(5):251–253.

Halper, J. (1990). The functional model in multiple sclerosis. *Rehabilitation Nursing, 15*(2):77–79, 85.

Holland, N. et al. (1988). A comparative study of impairment ratings in multiple sclerosis patients. *Rehabilitation Nursing, 13*(5):244–250.

Kassirer, M., and Osterberg, D. (1987). Pain in multiple sclerosis. *American Journal of Nursing, 87*:968–969.

Kelly, B., and Mahon, S. (1988). Nursing care of the patient with multiple sclerosis. *Rehabilitation Nursing, 13*(5):238–242.

Larson, P. (1990). Psychosocial adjustment in multiple sclerosis. *Rehabilitation Nursing, 15*(5):242–245.

Maloney, F., Burks, J., and Ringel, S. (1985). *Interdisciplinary rehabilitation of multiple sclerosis and neuromuscular disorders.* Philadelphia: J. B. Lippincott.

Marks, S., and Millard, R. (1990). Nursing assessment of positive adjustment for individuals with multiple sclerosis. *Rehabilitation Nursing, 15*(3):147–151.

Matthews, B. (1985). *Multiple sclerosis: The facts* (2nd ed.). New York: Oxford University Press.

McDonald, W., and Silberberg, D. (Eds.). (1986). *Multiple sclerosis.* Boston: Butterworths.

Schapiro, R. (1986). *Symptom management in multiple sclerosis.* New York: Demos Publications.

Scheinberg, L., and Holland, N. (Eds.). (1987). *Multiple sclerosis: A guide for patients and their families* (2nd ed.). New York: Raven Press.

Waksman, B., Reingold, S., and Reynolds, W. (1988). *Research on multiple sclerosis* (3rd ed.). New York: Demos Publications.

Walsh, P., and Walsh, A. (1987). Self-esteem and disease adaptation among multiple sclerosis patients. *Journal of Social Psychology, 127*(6):669–671.

Winters, S., Jackson, P., Sikms, K., and Magilvy, J. (1989). A nurse managed MS clinic: Improved quality of life for persons with MS. *Rehabilitation Nursing, 14*(1):13–16.

Amyotrophic Lateral Sclerosis Management

12

OBJECTIVES

After completing this chapter, the reader will be able to:

- Describe the pathophysiology of amyotrophic lateral sclerosis (ALS).
- Discuss the alterations in neuromuscular function associated with ALS.
- Describe the systemic complications that may develop with ALS and discuss preventive and treatment measures.
- Discuss methods to assist the patient in maintaining an optimal nutritional status.
- Describe interventions for maximizing the patient's functional potential.
- Discuss interventions to assist the patient and family in coping with the disability and prognosis.

INTRODUCTION

Amyotrophic lateral sclerosis (ALS) is a devastating degenerative disease of the upper and lower motor neurons of the CNS, with a very poor prognosis. It strikes 3 in every 100,000 people a year. The average age of onset is between 50 and 60 years. The male-female ratio is approximately 3 to 2. The ratio equalizes as women approach menopause. Because there is no known cure, individuals with ALS are faced with the overwhelming task of coping with progressive functional losses and a premature death. The patient and family need the expertise of rehabilitation nurses and other rehabilitation team members to help them deal competently with day-to-day management issues, to prevent complications, to maximize the quality of time the patient has, and to help them prepare for eventual death.

PATHOPHYSIOLOGY

Progressive upper and lower neuron degeneration is the primary pathological process with ALS. "Amyotrophic" refers to the muscle weakness and atrophy that result from the degeneration of the motor neurons in the anterior horn cells of the spinal cord, and in the motor nuclei of the cranial nerves (trigeminal V, facial VII, vagus X, spinal accessory XI, and hypoglossal XII). The neurons in the anterior horns of the second sacral segment are spared. "Lateral sclerosis" pertains to the demyelination and degeneration of the upper motor neurons in the corticospinal tract. Concurrent progression of the disease at all levels results in a combined picture of amyotrophy (lower motor neuron (LMN) involvement and spasticity (UMN involvement).

In 20 percent of the cases the course of ALS plateaus for extended periods of time, sometimes permanently. Fifty percent of persons with ALS die within 3 years of onset with 20 percent surviving beyond 5 years and 10 percent surviving beyond 10 years. The individuals with the shortest survival rate are those with bulbar involvement. Those persons with longer survival rates are most often those that have acquired the disease at a younger age and do not have bulbar involvement.

Complications

The respiratory complications of atelectasis, pneumonia, and respiratory failure are the primary causes of death in persons in ALS. These complications are usually the result of a combination of factors: Decreased mobility, dysphagia with aspiration, and respiratory lems early in the course of the disease. People with other types of ALS will experience these respiratory complications with increasing frequency as the disease progresses.

Some of the other potential complications that occur with ALS are related to the severity of the motor deficits and the degree of immobility and deconditioning. Therefore, the incidence of the following complications increases as the disease progresses:

- Cardiovascular: Deep vein thrombosis (DVT) and pulmonary embolism (PE), dependent edema.
- Urological: Urinary tract infection and calculi (urgency, frequency, or hesitancy may occur in late stages of the disease).
- Gastrointestinal: Constipation, impaction, nutritional deficits.
- Integumentary: Decubiti.
- Musculoskeletal: Contractures, falls.

Classification

There are three variants of the classical form of ALS.

Spinal muscular atrophy, related to lower motor neuron damage, presents a clinical picture of limb weakness and wasting with or without cranial nerve involvement. In some cases UMN symptoms may precede signs of LMN disease by long periods of time.

Progressive bulbar palsy, related to cranial motor neuron damage, is manifested by weakness and atrophy of the facial and oral muscles resulting in difficulty with speaking and swallowing. There may be atrophy and fasciculations of the tongue. The cough reflex may be hyperactive or greatly diminished. UMN changes in the brainstem may be associated with emotional lability and a hyperactive gag reflex.

Primary lateral sclerosis, related to upper motor neuron damage, is manifested by signs of spasticity and hyperactive deep tendon reflexes with no evidence of the muscle atrophy of LMN involvement. Because afferent nerves are intact the spasms are painful.

ALS is also classified according to the initial presenting symptoms. About one-third of the individuals with ALS have presenting symptoms of hand and finger weakness and difficulty performing fine motor tasks (brachial manual amyotrophy type). About one-third present with weakness in the lower extremities (crural type). In the remaining one-third the presenting complains include speech and swallowing difficulties (bulbar type).

Sinaki and Mulder (Scott, 1983) describe stages for assessing the overall level of an individual's disability: I. Ambulatory and independent with mild weakness; II. Has moderate weakness with upper extremity (UE) limitations; III. Ambulatory with severe UE limitations and moderate lower extremity (LE) limitations; IV. Confined to wheelchair but almost independent with severe LE involvement in mild UE involvement; V. In wheelchair and dependent with severe LE and moderate to severe UE involvement; and VI. Bedridden and totally dependent. Characteristically the disease progresses to involve all the muscles of the body, regardless of the initial onset site.

Theories of Etiology and Related Research Findings

While the etiology of ALS has been attributed to disorders of viral, toxic, metabolic, hereditary, ore immune origin, no definitive cause has been identified. Therapeutic trials with interferon and other antiviral substances have failed to alter the course of the disease. Though toxins and heavy metals such as mercury and lead have been implicated as causative factors, the majority of persons with ALS do not have toxic metal levels in the blood, urine, cerebrospinal fluid, or muscles.

The incidence of ALS is fairly evenly distributed throughout the world. However, clusters of individuals with ALS have been found in the Chamorro population on the island of Guam and in the inhabitants of western New Guinea and the Kii Peninsula of Japan. The water and soil in these three areas are low in calcium and magnesium and high in aluminum and manganese. Researchers suggest that these environmental conditions could lead to aberrant mineral metabolism with deposition of calcium, aluminum, and silicon in the motor neurons of the area's residents.

Another theory of metabolic dysfunction is supported by the evidence of impaired gluconate metabolism in persons with ALS. Gluconate is an amino acid involved with the transmission of nerve impulses. Two experimental treatments (the branched chain amino acid treatment and the L-threonine treatment) are designed to correct gluconate metabolic dysfunction. No conclusive results have yet been reported from these studies.

A familial tendency has been noted in 5 to 10 percent of the ALS population. Though an autosomal dominant pattern can be seen in this group, no specific genetic factor has been identified.

Detailed immunological screening of persons with ALS does not indicate a defect in immunoreactivity or immunoregulation. The removal of antibodies by plasmapheresis has been of no benefit in affecting the course of the disease. Studies are in process to determine whether total lymphoid irradiation or the administration of cyclosporine can slow or reverse the degenerative process.

NURSING INTERVENTIONS

Assessment

Health History

- Complains of generalized fatigue over a period of weeks to months.
- Complains of muscle cramping, weakness, and twitching of finger, hand, and arm muscles or feet and leg muscles over a period of weeks to months.
- Complains of difficulty performing fine motor tasks with fingers or difficulty in walking leading to falls.
- Complains of finger stiffness, later in hands and arms, or complains of feet stiffness, later in legs.
- Complains of swallowing difficulties with choking on fluids and foods.
- Complains of emotional lability.
- Pre-existing conditions or diseases.
- Current medication.
- Known allergies.
- Personal history including diet, sleep, smoking, and exercise patterns and psychosocial status.

Physical Assessment Findings

- Fasciculations of finger, hand, and arm muscles, later followed by weakness and atrophy of these muscles.
- Finger stiffness.
- Loss of fine motor abilities.
- Generalized hyper-reflexia.

- Intact sensation (though sensory involvement is rare, some individuals do experience paresthesias, tightness, pain and abnormalities of touch and pressure in the areas innervated by the peroneal and axonal nerves).
- Intact bowel and bladder function (urinary frequency, urgency or hesitancy in later stages).
- Fasciculations of foot and leg muscles later followed by weakness and atrophy of these muscles.
- Stiffness of feet and later of legs.
- Lower extremity spasticity.
- Weakness and atrophy of trunk and shoulder muscles.
- Weakness and atrophy of tongue, pharynx, larynx, and neck muscles.
- Intact cognitive functions.
- Emotional lability.

Diagnostic Tests

- Skull and spine x-rays to rule out bone deformities that may cause neurological manifestations.
- Myelogram and computed tomography (CT scan) to rule out other spinal cord pathology.
- Lumbar puncture to demonstrate normal pressure and to rule out possible infectious causes of neurological symptoms.
- Electromyography (EMG) and muscle biopsy to distinguish between myopathic and neurogenic disorders and between peripheral nerve damage and involvement of the anterior horn cells.
- EMG and nerve conduction studies that reveal the presence of widespread anterior horn cell dysfunction.
- Muscle biopsies that reveal atrophy of muscle fibers.
- Sensory tests that reveal no deficits.
- Tensilon test to rule out myasthenia gravis.
- Blood studies that reveal elevated acetylcholinesterase (ACHE), and creatinine phosphokinase (CPK).

There are no laboratory markers for ALS. Diagnosis is based on the recognition of a characteristic clinical profile which includes fatigue, muscle cramping and fasciculations, and progressive muscle weakness and atrophy.

Nursing Diagnoses: Actual or Potential

1. Impaired physical mobility related to muscle weakness, spasticity, pain.
2. Altered comfort: Pain related to cramping, stiffness, and spasticity.
3. Impaired communication related to motor deficits.
4. Potential for injury related to motor deficits
5. Self-care deficits related to motor deficits.
6. Activity intolerance related to pain, deconditioning, and/or motor deficits.
7. Altered tissue perfusion: Peripheral related to impaired venous circulation to extremities.
8. Respiratory dysfunction: Hypoventilation related to respiratory muscle weakness; pulmonary congestion related to aspiration and/or immobility.
9. Impaired skin integrity related to immobility, mechanical factors, altered nutritional status.
10. Altered bowel elimination: Constipation related to immobility, lack of privacy, inadequate diet.
11. Altered nutritional status: Less than body requirements related to anorexia, chewing/swallowing difficulties, inability to feed self.
12. Uncompensated swallowing impairment related to motor deficits.
13. Altered urinary elimination: Urgency, frequency, hesitation related to neurological dysfunction.
14. Sexual dysfunction related to biopsychosocial alteration of sexuality, absence of role models, lack of privacy, lack of knowledge.
15. Social isolation related to motor and communication deficits, environmental barriers.
16. Disturbance in self-concept: Body image, self-esteem.
17. Anxiety related to threat to self-concept, role functioning and interaction patterns; unmet needs, poor prognosis.
18. Grieving: Dysfunctional or anticipatory related to actual or perceived losses.
19. Ineffective individual or family coping related to inadequate information, inadequate support, multiple life changes.
20. Knowledge deficit related to ALS management.

Expected Outcomes: Patient and/or Family

1. The individual maintains functional alignment and sustains no complications of immobility.
2. The individual uses correct techniques to facilitate mobility and to compensate for motor deficits.
3. The individual is comfortable as evidenced by verbal statements and/or body language.
4. The individual employs an effective method of communication to convey thoughts and needs.
5. The individual remains free of injury.
6. The individual re-establishes role functions and socialization patterns and engages in self-care activities consistent with motor deficits and tolerance level.
7. The individual remains free of vascular complications.
8. The individual's lungs remain clear.
9. The individual's skin remains intact.
10. The individual's bowel and bladder patterns are stabilized.
11. The individual is free of urinary and bowel complications.
12. The individual maintains nutritional status as evidenced by stable body weight and normal hematocrit, hemoglobin, and serum protein.
13. The individual verbalizes perception of himself/herself as a sexual being.
14. The individual experiences decreased anxiety and improved self-concept as evidenced by verbal statements and/or body language.
15. The individual verbalizes and demonstrates an understanding of ALS management.

Planning and Implementation

(Include the family, significant other, and/or caregiver in the teaching interventions.)

Neurological Management

Administer medication as ordered to manage bulbar weakness (neostigmine bromide/Prostigmin). Observe and record the patient's response. Take measures to minimize side effects of the medications. Assist the patient in learning medication purpose, dosage, schedule, side effects, and precautions.

Assist the patient in learning pain relief measures such as relaxation exercises and self hypnosis to deal with painful spasticity and the discomforts of immobility. Avoid respiratory depressant pain medications. Administer medications as prescribed for painful cramping. Observe and record the patient's response. Take measures to minimize side effects of the medication. Assist the patient in learning the medication purpose, dosage, schedule, side effects, and precautions.

Assist the patient in learning the pathology, manifestations, and therapeutic management of ALS.

Communication Management

Encourage the patient to speak slowly and enunciate clearly. Reduce speaking anxiety by creating a relaxed, supportive, nonthreatening environment.

Work with the speech pathologist and occupational therapist to provide the patient with alternate communication methods as needed, such as a small computer with artificial speech articulation, a letter board, or an extra ocular controlled device.

Respiratory Management

Implement methods to maintain clear lungs and improve ventilation, such as coughing and deep breathing exercises, assistive coughing techniques, incentive spirometer, blow bottles, proper positioning, humidification, postural drainage, suctioning, and intermittent positive pressure breathing.

Assist the patient to maintain the maximum activity level possible.

Perform frequent respiratory assessments.

Provide the patient with additional respiratory support (oxygen, mechanical ventilation) as prescribed, using proper management techniques.

Protect the patient from temperature extremes and external sources of infection and respiratory irritants when possible.

Have standby suction equipment available.

Assist the patient and family in coping with the physical, psychological, and financial ramifications of progressive respiratory compromise.

Assist the patient in learning respiratory measures including positioning, chest therapy, signs and symptoms of complications, dysphagia management, and tracheostomy and ventilator care and suctioning, if applicable.

Cardiovascular Management

Implement measures to prevent DVT and PE and assist the patient in learning preventive measures. (See pages 143–144.)

Urological Management

Implement a bladder management program to prevent urinary tract complications related to decreased fluid intake and immobility. Assist the patient in learning prevention and treatment measures. (See pages 51–68.)

Gastrointestinal Management

Maintain adequate fluid intake and nutrition by monitoring the patient's weight, calorie and fluid intake, hemoglobin, hematocrit, and serum protein levels; working with the nutritionist to provide a high protein, balanced diet according to the patient's preferences; and working with the occupational therapist to provide adaptive eating aids as needed.

Minimize patient fatigue by providing small, more frequent feedings.

Provide mouth care after each meal to make sure no food that could be aspirated is still in the mouth.

Assist the patient in learning proper food selection, fluid and nutritional requirements, and safe eating/feeding techniques.

If dysphagia is present implement the appropriate management program. (See pages 81–92.)

Implement a bowel management program to prevent constipation. Assist the patient in learning prevention and treatment measures. (See pages 69–80.)

Integumentary Management

Implement measures to prevent skin breakdown. Assist the patient in learning preventive and treatment measures.

Musculoskeletal Management

Assist the patient to maximize functional potential, minimize spasticity, and prevent contractures. (See pages 148 and 150–151.)

Assist the patient in learning energy conservation methods and in the importance of avoiding temperature extremes.

Assist the patient in learning the safe and proper use of assistive devices and equipment such as motorized wheelchairs and portable ventilators.

Psychological Management

Explore the patient's feelings about the disease. Provide educational opportunities to increase his/her understanding of the condition and to increase his/her sense of control. Facilitate opportunities for peer interaction and sharing.

Assist the patient to regain self-confidence and a positive self-image by collaborating with him/her on realistic goal setting that capitalizes on personal strengths and resources. Promote the patient's self-esteem by providing positive feedback on learning and self-care efforts.

Provide family education to assist them in learning how to maximize the patient's independence and sense of worth.

Assist the patient and family in dealing with their stress and fears by encouraging them to share their feelings and fears, by providing them with referrals for individual counseling, and by assisting them in learning stress reduction techniques.

Refer the patient and family to community resources such as the ALS Association (15300 Ventura Boulevard, Sherman Oaks, CA 91403) for further support and information.

Sexuality Counseling

Assist the patient to maintain his/her sexual identity by minimizing the number of embarrassing and intrusive procedures and exposures, supporting the maintenance of physical appearance, acknowledging feelings and concerns, and facilitating the exploration of alternate or modified methods of sexual expression. (See pages 93–108.)

FUTURE IMPLICATIONS

ALS is a devastating disease with an unknown etiology and no known cure. Increased public awareness and funding can strengthen the research efforts that are directed toward finding the cause, effective preventive measures, and methods to prevent further motor neuron destruction once the disease has been acquired. Assisting the individual with ALS in maintaining health, independence, and an optimum quality of life are major challenges for nursing. Further studies are needed to discover additional physical and psychological intervention measures that will enhance the health, abilities, and physical and psychological comfort of all persons with ALS.

REFERENCES

Boss, B. (1988). The nervous system. In J. Howe, E. Dickason, D. Jones, & M. Snider (Eds.). *Handbook of Nursing.* New York: John Wiley and Sons.

Davis, R., and Robertson, D. (1985). *Textbook of neuropathology.* Baltimore: Williams and Wilkins.

Greene, C. (1987). *Handbook of adult primary care.* New York: John Wiley and Sons.

Hewer, R. (1988). Motor neuron disease. In Goodwill, J., and Chamberlain, A. *Rehabilitation of the physically disabled adult.* Dobbs Ferry, NY: Sheridan Medical Books, Sheridan House Inc.

Hickey, J. (1986). *The clinical practice of neurological and neurosurgical nursing* (2nd ed.). Philadelphia: J. B. Lippincott Company.

Mitsumoto, H., Hanson, M., and Chad, D. (1988). Amyotrophic lateral sclerosis: Recent advances in pathogenesis and therapeutic trials. *Archives of Neurology, 45*(2):189–202.

Nevins, S. (1986). The specific disorders affecting the central nervous system. In Kneisl, C., and Ames, S. *Adult health nursing: A biopsychoses.*

Pestronk, A., Adams, R., Clawson, L., Cornblath, D., Kunel, R., Griffin, D., and Drachman, D. (1988). Serum antibodies to GM_1 ganglioside in amyotrophic lateral sclerosis. *Neurology, 38*:1457–1461.

Scott, A. (1983). Degenerative diseases. In C. Trombly. *Occupational therapy for physical dysfunction* (2nd ed.). Baltimore: Williams and Wilkins.

Stone, N. (1987). ALS . . . A challenge for constant adaptation. *Journal of Neuroscience Nursing, 19*(3):166–173.

Parkinson's Disease Management

13

OBJECTIVES

After completing this chapter, the reader will be able to:

- Describe the pathophysiology of Parkinson's Disease (PD) and the related manifestations.
- Discuss the etiologies of parkinsonism.
- Describe two experimental treatment options for PD.
- Describe four common mobility impairments and the related management recommendations.
- Describe typical communication impairments and the related management recommendations.
- Discuss the categories of medication management for PD and describe the primary physiological and functional effects of each.
- Discuss interventions to enhance the patient's coping skills and facilitate psychosocial adjustment.

INTRODUCTION

Parkinson's Disease (PD) is a progressive, degenerative, neurological disorder affecting the brain centers responsible for control of movement. It is one of the most common nonvascular neurological disabilities and affects an estimated 1 million people in the United States. PD is characterized by a classic triad of symptoms: Muscular rigidity, nonintention tremor, and bradykinesia. Weakness, poverty

197

of movement, and balance problems and other characteristic manifestations.* The first symptoms most often appear in the sixth dec-
ade of life. Rehabilitation nurses working with individuals with PD
face the challenge of providing support and guidance that will enable patients to maximize functional potential while coping with
progressive losses and preventing complications related to these
losses.

PATHOPHYSIOLOGY

The complex of symptoms manifested in PD is reflective of dysfunction of the substantia nigra and the corpus striatum. Normally,
dopamine produced in the substantia nigra travels to the neurons of
the striatum where it exerts an excitatory effect. When the neurons
of the substantia nigra are injured, they cannot produce or store dopamine, resulting in a dopamine deficiency in the striatum. With a
severe deficiency, symptoms of parkinsonism appear. If the neurons
in the striatum that normally receive dopamine are damaged or the
action of dopamine is blocked, the effect is the same as that of a primary dopamine deficiency.

The course of PD is variable but usually has a slow steady progression over several years. The following scale was developed by
Hoehm and Yahr (O'Sullivan and Schmitz, 1988) as a means of recording an individual's degree of disability and the rate of disease
progression: Mild unilateral involvement, ADL independent—Stage
I; mild bilateral involvement, ADL independent—Stage II; moderate
bilateral disability, unsteadiness when turning or rising from chair,
some activities restricted but can live independently—Stage III; all
symptoms present and severe, requires help with some ADL—Stage
IV; totally disabled, confined to bed or wheelchair—Stage V.

Etiology

The majority of persons with parkinsonism manifestations have
some form of idiopathic degeneration related to the corpus striatum and the substantia nigra (idiopathic PD). However, similar dis-

---

*Parkinsonism refers not to a particular disease but to a condition with these charac-
teristic manifestations. PD is the most prevalent type of parkinsonism and remains
the prototype against which other types are compared.

orders of motor function can result from other pathological processes that impair these structures and/or the neurotransmitter system. Within this category are diseases such as encephalitis, atherosclerotic cerebrovascular disease, and neurosyphilis; exposure to carbon monoxide, manganese, or other toxic metals; and prolonged use of certain drugs such as fluphenazine hydrochloride (Prolixin), thioridazine hydrochloride (Mellaril), haloperidol (Haldol), mesoridazine (Serentil), and reserpine (Serpasil) that block the action of dopamine in the striatum.

Research

Research projects have been investigating causation theories as well as new medication and surgical interventions. One project in the preliminary stages is focusing on the trophic factors that can maintain or increase sprouting of dopamine neurons in the brain. One aspect of this project is to look at the effect of growth factors on fetal dopamine neurons in tissue culture to determine the promising ones that may benefit individuals with PD.

One new strategy for treatment is the use of NADH (nicotinamide adenine dinucleotide phosphate, reduced). Preliminary studies in Austria have demonstrated improvement in 75% of the people receiving NADH, though the exact mechanism of action is unclear. It is most effective in improving certain motor disabilities such as initiation of movement, gait, balance, and speech. It has little beneficial effect on tremor. It potentiates the effect of carbidopa/levodopa (Sinemet) and reduces the duration and severity of the "off" periods associated with levodopa therapy. No serious complications have been observed in these preliminary studies.

A surgical procedure that has received a great deal of publicity since 1987 is the transplantation of dopamine producing cells from the adrenal gland into the brain. Though improvement was reported in the selected candidates, the mortality rate was high. Further research is required to determine if this is in fact an effective procedure with sustained long-term improvement.

DATATOP is a NIH supported multicenter clinical trial investigating whether deprenyl (Eldepryl) and tocopherol (vitamin E) could slow the progression of PD. Initial results have shown deprenyl to be effective. The study is continuing to see how long it remains effective, to learn the mechanism of its effect, and to determine if tocopherol is also effective.

NURSING INTERVENTIONS

Assessment

Health History

- Complains of stiffness, slowness of movement, freezing episodes, stumbling, falling.
- Complains of mild, diffuse muscle pain.
- Complains of fatigue.
- Complains of excessive sweating and heat intolerance.
- Complains of urinary frequency and urgency and constipation.
- Complains of faintness and dizziness on sitting up and standing.
- Complains of depression.
- History of viral encephalitis or carbon monoxide, manganese, or other metallic poisoning or CNS trauma.
- Other pre-existing diseases or conditions.
- Current intake of tranquilizers/antipsychotic drugs and other medications.
- Known allergies.
- Personal history including diet, sleep, smoking, and exercise patterns and psychosocial history.

Physical Findings

Nonintention tremor

1. Ceasing with voluntary movement and when patient is sleeping.
2. Worse when patient is nervous, frightened, or angry.
3. Often one of the first manifestations of PD is pill-rolling motion of thumb against fingers, later tremor is seen in arms, jaw, eyelids, and feet.

Mobility impairments

1. Bradykinesia.
2. Akinesia.
3. Difficulty starting and stopping movement.

4. Festinating gait.
5. Propulsive gait.
6. Freezing.
7. Dyskinesia.
8. Increasing rigidity with presence of cogwheel phenomena during passive motions.
9. Loss of automatic associated movement such as loss of arm swing when walking.
10. Impaired handwriting.

Postural and reflex changes

1. Hypertonias in flexor muscles in trunk and extremities resulting in stooped posture with arms at sides, elbows flexed, fingers abducted and flexed.
2. Loss of postural and balancing reflexes.
3. Mask-like facial expression and reduced blinking.

Speech impairments

1. Difficulty initiating speech.
2. Difficulty in coordinating expiration and articulation.
3. Low pitched voice becoming only a whisper or inaudible over time.
4. Lack of modulation.
5. Dysarthria.

Dysphagia
Urinary frequency and urgency
Autonomic effects

1. Increased lacrimation and sialorrhea.
2. Orthostatic hypotension.
3. Sebarrhea and diaphoresis.

Cognitive dysfunctions

1. Short-term memory loss.
2. Short attention span.
3. Bradyphrenia.
4. Dementia (may be seen in advanced PD).

Diagnostic Tests

Electroencephalogram revealing brain wave abnormalities.

Serum blood studies to rule out endocrine and metabolic disorders or toxic states.

Lumbar puncture to rule out abnormal cerebrospinal fluid pressure and analysis.

Computed tomography (CT Scan) to rule out bleeding, hydrocephalus, tumor, or other mass lesions.

Positron emission tomography (PET Scan) to demonstrate characteristic changes in brain metabolism.

Nursing Diagnosis: Actual or Potential

1. Impaired cognition related to short-term memory and problem-solving deficits.
2. Impaired physical mobility related to muscle rigidity, tremor, bradykinesia, flexion posturing, loss of postural reflexes.
3. Altered comfort: Aching and muscle cramping related to rigidity and flexion posturing.
4. Impaired verbal communication: Soft and monotonous voice related to motor deficits.
5. Self-care deficit: Feeding, bathing/hygiene, dressing/grooming, toileting related to motor and/or cognitive deficits, pain, fatigue, depression.
6. Potential for injury related to motor, and/or cognitive deficits.
7. Respiratory dysfunction: Pulmonary congestion and atelectasis related to immobility; aspiration related to dysphagia; impaired ventilation related to muscle rigidity.
8. Impaired skin integrity related to immobility, excessive sweating, altered nutritional status.
9. Altered bowel elimination: Constipation related to immobility, inadequate diet, medication side effects.
10. Altered nutritional status: Less than body requirements related to chewing/swallowing difficulties, inability to feed self.
11. Uncompensated swallowing impairment related to motor deficits.
12. Altered urinary elimination: Urgency and frequency related

to neurological dysfunction; hesitancy, retention related to medication side effects.

13. Social isolation related to communication barriers, self-concept disturbances, limited mobility, environmental barriers, cognitive impairments.
14. Sexual dysfunction related to biopsychosocial alteration of sexuality, absence of role models, lack of privacy, lack of knowledge.
15. Disturbance in self-concept: Body image, self-esteem.
16. Anxiety related to threat to self-concept, role functioning and interaction patterns; unmet needs.
17. Grieving: Dysfunctional or anticipatory related to actual or perceived losses.
18. Ineffective individual or family coping related to inadequate information, inadequate support, multiple life changes.
19. Knowledge deficit related to Parkinson's disease management.

Expected Outcomes

1. The individual maintains cognitive abilities.
2. The individual maintains functional alignment and sustains no complication of immobility.
3. The individual uses correct techniques to facilitate mobility and to compensate for motor deficits.
4. The individual is comfortable as evidenced by verbal statements and/or body language.
5. The individual employs an effective method of communication to convey thoughts and needs.
6. The individual reestablishes role functions and socialization patterns and engages in self-care activities consistent with motor deficits and tolerance level.
7. The individual remains free of injury.
8. The individual's lungs remain clear.
9. The individual's skin remains intact.
10. The individual is free of urinary and bowel complications.
11. The individual's bowel and bladder patterns are stabilized.
12. The individual maintains nutritional status as evidenced by stable body weight and normal hematocrit, hemoglobin, and serum protein.

13. The individual verbalizes perception of himself/herself as a sexual being.
14. The individual experiences decreased anxiety and improved self-concept as evidenced by verbal statements and/or body language.
15. The individual verbalizes and demonstrates an understanding of PD management.

Planning and Implementation

(Include the family, significant other, and/or caregiver in the teaching interventions.)

Mobility Management

To prevent stiffness and contractures and to maintain posture, work with physical and occupational therapy to maintain a program of stretching, range of motion, and postural exercises. Assist the patient with warm baths/showers to relax muscles and relieve painful spasms. Encourage him/her to sleep on a firm mattress without a pillow to prevent head flexion.

To avoid freezing when confronted with minor obstacles, encourage the patient to concentrate on taking large steps, lifting feet high, and taking the hand or arm of a helper for gentle support. If a freezing episode occurs, instruct the individual to raise head and toes and rock from one foot to the other while bending knees slightly. Other suggestions for overcoming freezing episodes include asking the individual to raise his/her arms in a sudden short motion, to take a small step backward then start forward, or to step sideways then start forward. Instruct the family not to pull the patient during a freezing episode as this increases the problem and may cause falling.

To overcome the patient's fear of falling, encourage him/her to touch the ground with heel first and lift the toes with each step; grasp hands behind the back when walking and keep feet wide apart for better balance and posture; make turns with series of small steps rather than crossing legs over.

To overcome variations in ability to move encourage the patient to maintain a consistent activity schedule with frequent short walks and other activities involving moderate movement. Discuss the advisability of scheduled rest periods to avoid overtiring.

To facilitate rising from a chair, encourage the patient to use a straight backed wooden chair with arms and a two-inch elevation added to the back legs of the chair to give a slight forward tilt; then, when attempting to rise, the patient should move toward the edge of the seat, placing his/her heels as far back under the chair as possible, leaning forward from the hips so that the center of gravity is above the feet before rising to a standing position.

Assist the patient in learning the use of assistive and supportive devices and, in general, safety measures to protect from injury related to mobility impairments.

To help control excessive tremor of the hands and arms, encourage the patient to sit in a chair and grasp the chair arms.

Communication and Cognitive Management

Work with the speech pathologist on a program to improve the patient's communication abilities. Encourage the individual to exaggerate pronunciation; take a breath before speaking, and pause between every few words; express ideas in short concise phrases; take time to organize thoughts before speaking; and face listener when speaking. Encourage the use of communication aids prescribed by the speech pathologist, such as a voice amplifier.

Refer to pages 124–125 for management of memory and problem-solving deficits. Assist the patient in learning safety measures to prevent injury related to cognitive impairments.

Respiratory Management

To prevent choking and aspiration related to dysphagia, institute a dysphagia management program. (See pages 81–92.)

To prevent choking and aspiration related to excess salivation and impaired cough mechanism, encourage the patient to make a conscious effort to swallow frequently; maintain head in an upright position so saliva will collect in the back of the throat and facilitate automatic swallowing; sleep in a prone or sidelying position.

Work with the respiratory therapist and patient on a program of breathing exercises to mobilize the rib cage and improve aeration of the lungs.

Assist the patient in learning dysphagia management, positioning, respiratory exercises, and the proper use of suctioning equipment.

Integumentary Management

Implement measures to prevent skin breakdown. Assist the patient in learning preventive and treatment measures. (See pages 146–148.)

Gastrointestinal Management

To maintain adequate nutritional and fluid intake, work with the dietician to implement an individualized nutritional support program. Institute a dysphagia management program when indicated.

To prevent constipation resulting from decreased mobility, autonomic dysfunction, and anticholinergic medication, implement a bowel management program.

Assist the patient in learning preventive and treatment measures. (See pages 69–80.)

Medication Management

Pharmacological treatment is primarily focused on the attempt to restore dopamine to normal levels in the CNS (specifically in the nigrostriatal system). Drug choices are based in part on the most prominent clinical manifestations exhibited by the patient. Drug therapy decreases but does not halt the progression of the disease and requires ongoing adjustments as the disease progresses. The following medications or medication groups are those most often prescribed to treat PD.

I. Dopaminergic

A. Levodopa (L-Dopa, Dopar, Larodopa)
   1. Converted to dopamine in the brain.
   2. Given in increasing doses until the patient's tolerance is reached.
   3. May take weeks or months for the effects to be seen.
   4. Clinical fluctuations in effectiveness frequently encountered (on-off phenomena).
   5. Increased patient tolerance & decreased drug effectiveness occurs with prolonged use.
   6. Relieves muscle rigidity in the majority of users and usually improves tremor for a period of time.
   7. Protein, vitamin B6 (pyridoxine), multivitamins, and alcohol may interfere with drug's effectiveness.
B. Carbidopa/levodopa (Sinemet)
   1. Inhibits use of dopamine outside of brain allowing more availability in the brain.
   2. Decreases the amount of levodopa needed by potentiating its therapeutic effect.

C. Amantadine hydrochloride (Symmetrel)
   1. Antiviral drug that may increase the release of dopamine in the brain.
   2. Moderately effective for all symptoms.
   3. Benefits may decrease after 3 to 6 months.
D. Deprenyl (Eldepryl)
   1. Prevents dopamine catabolism in the brain due to its enzymatic action.
   2. Used in early stages of PD as first line of defense, later on is combined with other anti-PD drugs.

II. Dopamine agonists

A. Bromocriptine (Parlodel)
   1. Crosses blood brain barrier and stimulates dopanergic receptors.
   2. Used in early stages as primary treatment or later in combination with levodopa or Sinemet.
   3. Most useful in decreasing movement fluctuations.
B. Pergolide (Permax)
   1. More potent than bromocriptine.
   2. Particularly effective for PD related speech difficulties.

III. Antihistamines

A. Such as diphenhydramine hydrochloride (Benadryl) and chlorpheniramine maleate (Chlortrimeton)
   1. Occasionally helpful for mild tremor in clients with minimal dysfunction.

IV. Anticholinergics

A. Such as trihexphenidyl (Artane), cyrimine hydrochloride (Pagitane), benztropine mesylate (Cogentin), ethopropazine (Parsidol), biperiden (Akineton)
   1. Augment levodopa by blocking cholinergic receptors in the brain.
   2. May decrease tremor and rigidity and control drooling.
   3. Prescribed in early stages or later as adjunct therapy.

To temporarily eliminate or reduce symptom severity, administer medications as prescribed by the physician. Observe and record the patient's response. Assist the patient in learning the medication purpose, dosage, schedule, side effects, precautions, and special instructions.

To minimize side effects, instruct the patient to take dopaminergic medications with meals to diminish gastric irritation and nausea; to chew gum and suck on hard candy to reduce mouth dryness associated with dopaminergic and anticholinergic medications; to rise slowly from a lying or sitting position, avoid standing still, and wear elastic stockings to reduce the orthostatic hypotension associated with dopaminergic medications; to follow the recommended bowel and bladder routines to avoid the constipation and urinary retention associated with dopaminergic and anticholinergic medications; to observe safety precautions to prevent injury as a result of the confusion and hallucinations associated with the dopamine agonists. Advise the patient that routine blood work and tonometry (screening test for glaucoma) may be ordered as levodopa and Sinemet can cause GI bleeding and exacerbate blood disorders and glaucoma.

Parkinsonian Crisis

Parkinsonian crisis is a condition resulting from the abrupt discontinuation of medication and/or psychological trauma. It is characterized by fever and a sudden, severe exacerbation of tremor, rigidity, and dyskinesia.

To manage parkinsonian crisis, control fever with antipyretic measures; resume medication schedules and administer intravenous or intramuscular phenobarbital as prescribed; provide a calm, quiet, supportive environment.

Surgical Management

Stereotaxic surgery is the creation of lesions in or destruction of portions of the globus pallidus, ventrolateral nucleus of the thalamus or the lenticular nuclei with electrocoagulation or cryosurgery. About 10 percent of patients with PD are selected for and benefit from this type of surgery (younger patients with predominantly one-sided tremor and rigidity that interferes with function despite medication therapy).

Provide pre- and post-op care as ordered. Prepare the patient and family for the surgery and what to expect in post-op management.

Psychological Management

To reduce depression and anxiety and improve coping abilities, assist the patient in establishing achievable goals; encourage him/ her to actively participate in therapy, social, and recreational events, and in structured group programs; provide a planned program of activity throughout the day. Help the patient identify problem areas and explore alternative methods of coping. Assist him/her in learning relaxation techniques. Provide counseling referral when indicated.

Promote self-esteem by providing positive feedback on learning and participation efforts.

Administer tricyclic antidepressant medication as ordered. Observe and record the patient's response. Assist the patient in learning medication purpose, dosage, schedule, side effects, and precautions.

Refer the patient and family to resource groups such as the American Parkinson Disease Association (116 John Street, Suite 417, New York, NY 10038-9982) and the Parkinson's Disease Foundation (650 West 168 Street, New York, NY 10032).

Sexuality Counseling

Assist the patient to maintain his/her sexual identity by minimizing the number of embarrassing and intrusive procedures and exposures; supporting the maintenance of physical appearance; acknowledging feelings and concerns; and facilitating the exploration of alternate or modified methods of sexual expression. (See pages 93–108.)

FUTURE IMPLICATIONS

In recent years advancements in medication management have helped control the symptoms of PD more effectively. Research studies are currently exploring the possibilities of medications that not only control symptoms but slow or reverse the progression of the disease. Other new treatments, such as the autologous transplantation of adrenal tissue and fetal transplantation, offer additional hope to persons with PD. In addition to the promises of ongoing research and advanced technology, the quality of each individual's life in relation to physical functioning and emotional health is most personally affected by the teaching, care, and support received from the rehabilitation nurses and other members of the rehabilitation team.

REFERENCES

Fahn, S. (1989). Adverse effects of levodopa in Parkinson's Disease. In D. Calne (Ed.). *Drugs for the treatment of Parkinson's Disease*. Berlin: Springer-Verlag.

Fahn, S. (1989). Involuntary movements. In L. Rowland (Ed.). *Merritt's Textbook of Neurology* (8th ed.). Philadelphia: Lea and Feiger.

Fahn, S. (1989). Parkinson's Disease and disorders with Parkinsonian features. In J. Hurst (Ed.). *Criteria for Diagnosis*. Boston: Butterworths.

Fahn, S., and Jankovic, J. (Eds.). (1989). Extrapyramidal, developmental, and inherited CNS disease. *Neurology Neurosurgery, 2*:303–352.

Fahn S., Marsden, D., Jenner, P., and Teychenne, P. (Eds.). (1986). *Recent developments in Parkinson's Disease*. New York: Raven Press.

Fahn, S., Marsden, D., Calne, D., and Goldsten, M. (Eds.). (1987). *Recent developments in Parkinson's Disease volume II*. Florham Park, NJ: Macmilliam Healthcare Information.

Godwin-Austen, R. (1989). *Parkinson's Disease handbook*. Baltimore: International Health.

Lang, A., and Fahn, S. (1989). Assessment of Parkinson's Disease. In T. Munsat (Ed.). *Quantification of neurologic deficit*. Boston: Butterworths.

Mayeux, R. (1989). A current analysis of behavioral problems in patients with idiopathic Parkinson's Disease. *Movement Disorders* (Supplement 1), 4:26–37.

Mitchell, P. (1987). Group exercises: A nursing therapy in Parkinson's Disease. *Rehabilitation Nursing, 12*(5):242–245.

O'Sullivan, S., and Schmitz, T. (1988). *Physical rehabilitation: Assessment and treatment* (2nd ed.). Philadelphia: F. A. Davis Company.

Palmer, S., Mortimer, J., Webster, D., Bistevins, R., and Dickinson, G. (1986). Exercise therapy in Parkinson's Disease. *Archives of Physical Medicine and Rehabilitation, 67*:741–745.

Parkinson Study Group. (1989). DATATOP: A multicenter controlled clinical trial in early Parkinson's Disease. *Archives of Neurology, 46*:1052–1060.

Parkinson Study Group. (1989). Effect of deprenyl on the progression of disability in early Parkinson's Disease. *New England Journal of Medicine, 321*:1364–1371.

Glossary

acalculia: inability to do simple arithmetic

agnosia: inability to recognize familiar objects through sense of sight, touch, or sound

agraphia: inability to express thoughts in writing

akinesia: general weakness and poverty of movement

alexia: inability to read (with or without aphasia)

amaurosis fugax: temporary loss of vision from diminished blood flow to brain

amyotrophy: muscle wasting

anomia: inability to remember names of objects

anosognosia: severe form of neglect in which individual ignores a part of his/her body

anterograde amnesia: difficulty retaining information after TBI; difficulty with new learning

aphasia: impairment in the ability to understand and produce language (see fluent, global, and nonfluent aphasia)

aphonia: inability to produce speech sounds from larynx

apraxias: disorders of programming resulting in inability to perform purposive movements, to use objects correctly, or to remember orders and instructions

areflexic: without reflexes

association: ability to make a connection between ideas, perceptions

asteroeognosia: inability to recognize objects or forms by touch

asthenia: lack of strength

ataxia: muscular incoordination

autonomic hyperreflexia (dysreflexia): exaggerated sympathetic response to noxious stimuli below level of spinal cord injury

bradykinesia: slowness of movement

bradyphrenia: slowness in thinking

categorization: ability to correctly classify information

circumlocution: indirect, evasive speech

cognition: ability to comprehend and process information

coma: period of prolonged unconsciousness and unresponsiveness to environment

concussion: transient neurological dysfunction with brief loss of consciousness

confabulation: verbalization which reflects confused thinking

confused language: characterized by faulty memory, unclear thinking, disorientation, irrelevance, and confabulation

contre-coup: damage to the brain opposite the site of impact

contusion: bruising or crushing injury to brain with loss of consciousness of varying lengths of time

cortical blindness: resulting from a lesion of visual area of cortex

coup: damage to the brain at point of impact

disinhibition: inability to control or inhibit impulses and emotions

detrusor sphincter dyssynergia: incoordination between bladder and sphincter

dysarthria: distorted, slurred speech production related to neuromuscular dysfunction

dysgraphia: impairment in writing ability due to language deficit

dyskinesia: jerky, uncoordinated, involuntary movement

dyslexia: impairment in reading ability due to language deficit

dysmetria: failure to stop movements correctly

dysphagia: difficulty in swallowing related to neuromuscular dysfunction

dysreflexia (autonomic hyperreflexia): exaggerated sympathetic response to noxious stimuli below level of spinal cord injury

echolalia: involuntary, parrot-like repetition of words spoken by others

extrapyramidal: relating to the basal ganglia

festinating gait: shuffling gait with little steps (petitepes)

fluent aphasia (receptive, sensory, Wernicke's): verbal expression characterized by quantity of verbal output with circumlocution, paraphasia, jargon, abnormal comprehension

freezing: unpredictable gait interruption

global aphasia: defective verbal expression, comprehension, writing, and reading

hematoma: a swelling or mass of blood caused by blood vessel damage

heterotopic ossification: a condition where calcium is lost from bones and deposited in skeletal muscles and tendons (myositis ossificans) or around joints (peri-articular ossification)

homonymous hemianopsia: loss of visual field in nasal half of one eye and temporal half of the other

hydronephrosis: dilation of upper urinary tract

hyperalgesia: increased sensitivity of pain receptors on pathologic conditions

hyperesthesia: unusual sensitivity to sensory stimuli

hyperreflexic: spastic, hypertonic

hypesthesia: diminished sensation

intercalated neuron: neuron between the afferent and efferent neurons of a reflex arc

lability: loss of emotional control, usually manifested by excessive and/or inappropriate laughter or crying

Lhermitte's sign: associated with MS; sensation of electric shock which extends down arms and back when neck flexed

lower motor neuron lesion: injury below L1 characterized by a flaccid paralysis

micrographia: progressively smaller handwriting

neurogenic bladder or bowel: impaired function of these organs resulting from interference in central or peripheral nervous system

nonfluent aphasia (expressive, motor, Broca's): verbal expression characterized by decreased output and increased effort of delivery, comprehension may be normal or abnormal

nystagmus: constant, involuntary movement of eyeball

opthmoplegia: paralysis of ocular muscles

paraparesis: weakness of lower extremities

paraplegia: paralysis of lower extremities

paraphasia: substitutions within a syllable or word

paresthesia: abnormal sensation without objective cause

parkinsonism: motor impairments resembling those of Parkinson's disease

perception: interpretation and integration of sensory stimuli from within the individual and from the environment

poikilothermic: varying according to environmental temperature

post traumatic amnesia: anterograde amnesia

proprioception: sense of the movement and position of body parts

propulsive gait: tendency to accelerate and fall forward with difficulty stopping

prosody abnormalities: difficulty with metrical structuring of language

quadriparesis: weakness of all four extremities

quadriplegia: paralysis of all four extremities

reflex arc: neural pathway between point of stimulation and responding organ in a reflex action

retrograde amnesia: inability to recall events prior to injury accident

retropulsion: tendency to accelerate backward

scanning speech: slow, hesitant speech characteristic of MS

scotomata: blind area in the visual field

seriation: ability to maintain continuous, sequential thought patterns

shunt: a procedure/device to drain off excessive cerebrospinal fluid in the brain

sialorrhea: excessive flow of saliva

somatognosia: lack of awareness of body structure and failure to recognize body parts in relationship

synthesis: ability to bring together separate thoughts into a unified whole

tactile defensiveness: heightened sense of touch

tangentiality: to suddenly break off one train of thought to pursue another

Ulthoff's phenomena: condition associated with MS in which weakness becomes worse after exposure to heat

upper motor neuron lesion: spinal cord lesion above L2 resulting in a hypertonic paralysis

unilateral neglect: inability to integrate and use perceptions from one side of body or environment

urolithiasis: formation of urinary calculi

vesicoureteric reflux: condition where urine backs up ureters

Psychological and Discharge Planning References

This list of references provides a starting point for a more indepth exploration of the psychology of rehabilitation, the family's role in rehabilitation, and discharge planning. The reference list at the end of each chapter includes more disability-specific references on these topics.

Ben-Sira, Z. (1986). Disability, stress, and readjustment: The function of the professional's latent goals and affective behavior in rehabilitation. *Social Science and Medicine, 23.*

Caplan, B. (1987). *Rehabilitation psychologic desk reference.* Rockville, MD: Aspen Publishers.

De Rienzo, B. (1985). Discharge planning. *Rehabilitation Nursing, 10*(4):34–36.

Evenson, T., Evenson, N., and Fish, D. (1986). Family enrichment: Rehabilitation opportunity. *Rehabilitation Literature, 47*:274–79.

Grant, J. and Bean, C. (1988). Stress: An analysis and application in rehabilitation nursing. *Rehabilitation Nursing, 13*(4):181–188.

Kolevzon, M. and Green, R. (1985). *Family therapy models: Convergence and divergence.* New York: Springer Publishing Company.

Mandel, A. and Keller, S. (1986). Stress management in rehabilitation. *Archives of Physical Medicine and Rehabilitation, 67*:375–379.

Marinelli, R. and Dell Orto, A. (1984). The psychological and social impact of physical disability (2nd ed.). New York: Springer Publishing Company.

McNett, S. (1987). Social support, threat, and coping responses and effectiveness in the functionally disabled. *Nursing Research, 36*:98–103.

Mumma, C. (Ed.) (1987). Theoretical background. In Mumma, C. (Ed.). *Re-*

habilitation nursing: Concepts and practice (2nd ed.). Evanston, IL: Rehabilitation Nursing Foundation.

Naugle, R. (1988). Denial in rehabilitation: Its genesis and clinical management. *Rehabilitation Counseling Bulletin, 31*:218–231.

Patrick, D., Morgan, M., and Charlton, J. (1986). Psychosocial support and change in the health status of physically disabled people. *Social Science and Medicine, 22*:1347–1354.

Pollock, S. (1986). Human responses to chronic illness: Physiologic and psychosocial adaptation. *Nursing Research, 35*:90–95.

Power, P. (1989). Working with females: An intervention model for rehabilitation nurses. *Rehabilitation Nursing, 14*(2):73–76.

Power, P., Dell Orto, A., and Gibbons, M. (Eds.) (1988). *Family interventions throughout chronic illness and disability.* New York: Springer Publishing Company.

Rosenbaum, M. (Ed.) (1990). *Learned resourcefulness: On coping skills, self control, and adaptive behavior.* New York: Springer Publishing Company.

Sutton, J. (1985). The need for family involvement in client rehabilitation. *Journal of Applied Rehabilitation Counseling, 16*:42–45.

Van de Bittner, S. (Ed.) (1987). Reintegration of the client into the community. In Mumma, C. (Ed.). *Rehabilitation nursing: Concepts and practice* (2nd ed.). Evanston, IL: Rehabilitation Nursing Foundation.

Vash, C. (1981). *The psychology of disability.* New York: Springer Publishing Company.

White, M. and Holloway, M. (1990). Patient concerns after discharge from rehabilitation. *Rehabilitation Nursing, 15*(6):316–318.

Wright, B. (1983). *Physical disability: A psychosocial approach.* New York: Harper and Row.

Resource Phone Numbers

The following organizations (telephone numbers included) provide information on disability-related concerns.

Accent On Information, (309) 378-2961

Advocacy Center for the Elderly and Disabled, (800) 662-7705

American Coalition of Citizens with Disability, (202) 628-3470

American Heart Association, (214) 373-6300

American Paralysis Association, (800) 225-0292, (201) 379-2690

American Parkinson's Disease Association, (800) 223-2732

American Speech, Language, and Hearing Association,
    (800) 638-8255

Amyotrophic Lateral Sclerosis Association, (800) 782-4747,
    (813) 340-7500

Association for Advancement of Rehabilitation Technology,
    (202) 857-1199

AT&T Office on Devices for People with Disabilities, (800) 233-1222

AT&T Special Needs Center, (800) 833-3232

Center for Health Promotion and Education Hotline,
    (404) 329-3492

Center for Rehabilitation Technology Hotline, (404) 894-4960

Clearing House for the Handicapped, (202) 730-1245

Disability Rights Center, (202) 223-3304

ERIC Clearinghouse on Adult Career and Vocational Education, (800) 848-4815

HEATH (Higher Education and Adult Training for People with Handicaps), (800) 544-3248, (202) 939-9320

IBM National Support Center for Persons with Disabilities, (800) 526-2133

Independent Community Assistance Network, (800) 654-6153

Independent Living Research Utilization, (713) 797-0200

Information Center for Individuals with Disabilities, (617) 727-5540

Inspector General's Hotline Department of Health and Human Services, (800) 368-5779, (301) 597-0724

Institute for Rehabilitation Disability Management, (202) 547-6644

Medicare Medicaid Complaint Line, (800) 368-5779, (301) 597-0724

Miami Project to Cure Paralysis, (800) 782-6387

National Association for Hearing and Speech Action, (800) 638-8255

National Association of Medical Equipment Suppliers, (703) 836-6263

National Association of the Physically Handicapped, (614) 852-1664

National Association of Rehabilitation Facilities, (703) 556-8848, (301) 654-5882

National Council of the Handicapped, (202) 453-3846

National Council of Independent Living Programs, (312) 225-5900

National Easter Seal Society, (800) 221-6827

National Handicapped Sports and Recreation Association, (301) 652-7505

National Head Injury Foundation, (800) 262-9500, (800) 444-6443, (508) 485-9950

National Health Information Clearinghouse, (800) 836-4797, (703) 522-5290

National Health Information Center Hotline, (800) 336-4797

National Information Center for Children and Youth with Handicaps, (800) 999-5599

National Injury Information Clearinghouse Hotline, (301) 492-6424

National Institute of Communicative Disorders and Stroke Hotline, (301) 496-5924

National Institutes of Health, (301) 496-5751

National Library Services for the Blind and Physically Handicapped, (202) 287-5100

National Multiple Sclerosis Society, (800) 624-8236

National Organization on Disability, (202) 293-5960

National Parkinson Foundation, (800) 327-4545, (305) 547-6666

National Paraplegic Foundation, (312) 346-4779

National Rehabilitation Association, (703) 836-0850

National Rehabilitation Information Center, (800) 346-2742

National Spinal Cord Injury Association, (800) 962-9629

National Spinal Cord Injury Hotline, (800) 526-3456, (800) 962-9629

National Wheelchair Athletic Association, (303) 632-0698

Paralyzed Veterans of America, (800) 232-1782, (202) 872-1300

Parkinson's Educational Program, (800) 344-7872, (714) 640-0218

President's Committee on Employment of the Handicapped Hotline (202) 653-5044

Rehabilitation Services Administration Department of Education, (202) 732-1282

Research and Training Center on Independent Living, (913) 842-7694

SERIES (Special Education and Rehabilitation Extension System), (800) 356-3269, (503) 346-3534

Society for the Advancement of Travel for the Handicapped, (718) 858-5483

Spinal Network, (800) 338-5412

Stifel Paralysis Research Foundation, (800) 225-0292.

United Organization of Persons with Disabilities, (602) 882-5476

United States Department of Education, (800) 848-4815

World Institute on Disability, (415) 486-8314

Index